"Grabovac and Cayoun are true masters of mindfulness and meditation, and in particular the clinical implementation of insight and related psychological and philosophical constructs. With this workbook, they provide an extremely powerful tool for working with negative mood and anxiety that promises to facilitate deep, meaningful, and real healing for the benefit of many."

> —**Matthew D. Sacchet, PhD**, associate professor and director of the Meditation Research Program in the department of psychiatry at Massachusetts General Hospital, Harvard Medical School

"This exceptional book, written by seasoned experts, harmoniously integrates Buddhist psychology and cognitive behavioral therapy (CBT) to effectively address depression and anxiety. It offers a systematic process that guides readers on a journey of self-discovery, empowering them to reclaim mental control, reduce reactivity, overcome avoidance, foster confidence in relationships, and minimize relapse risks."

> —**Susan Woods, MSW**, coauthor of *Mindfulness-Based Cognitive Therapy* and *Mindfulness-Based Stress Reduction*

"Grabovac and Cayoun's workbook provides an exceptional framework for understanding and managing mental health. By integrating mindfulness with cognitive behavioral strategies, this guide empowers individuals to regain control over their thoughts and emotions. Through gradual exposure to overcome avoidance, enhancing interpersonal skills for empathetic communication, and fostering compassion and equanimity, it's an essential guide for anyone looking to reclaim their life from anxiety and depression while fostering a profound sense of agency and peace."

> —**Lic. María Noel Anchorena**, clinical psychologist, professor, certified mindfulness-based stress reduction (MBSR) teacher and teacher trainer, and cofounder and general director at Sociedad Mindfulness y Salud

"This is a beautiful book. Andrea D. Grabovac and Bruno A. Cayoun have a distinctive voice within the mindfulness field for which they are known internationally. Here you will discover how ancient wisdom teachings—combined skillfully with modern psychological approaches—can offer healing for the mental and physical pain created by anxiety and depression that seems overwhelming. Allow yourself to be guided step by step through their clinically proven mindfulness program, remaining open in heart and mind, and you will find practices that will bring freedom in new and surprising ways."

> —**Mark Williams**, emeritus professor of clinical psychology at the University of Oxford, and coauthor of *Deeper Mindfulness*

"People managing a mood or anxiety disorder require a variety of tools to help them achieve emotional balance—this workbook provides exactly that. Its skillful interweaving of mindfulness practices and cognitive therapy exercises allows the reader to glide effortlessly between proven strategies for working with negative affect that lead to synergistic benefits and durable change."

—**Zindel V. Segal, PhD**, professor at the University of Toronto Scarborough, and coauthor of *Better in Every Sense*

"This workbook is a must for any person struggling with anxiety and/or depression. Grabovac and Cayoun are your personal therapists and meditation teachers holding your hand as you work through the MiCBT treatment, and their gentle voices are guiding you through the mindfulness practices. This workbook is an interactive experience with ample places for the reader to share their thoughts and emotions, their personal stories, and many suggestions for how to overcome roadblocks."

—**Lori A. Brotto, PhD**, professor at the University of British Columbia, and author of *Better Sex Through Mindfulness*

"A thoughtful and comprehensive workbook that combines mindfulness and cognitive behavioral techniques to provide effective strategies for managing anxiety and depression. The structured program and practical exercises make it an accessible and effective tool for anyone seeking mental health and well-being. A valuable resource for both individuals and therapists."

—**Nicholas T. Van Dam, PhD**, associate professor of psychological sciences, and inaugural director of the Contemplative Studies Centre at The University of Melbourne

# Mindfulness and Meditation

## Workbook for Anxiety and Depression

Balance Emotions, Overcome Intrusive Thoughts,
and Find Peace Using **Mindfulness-integrated CBT**

ANDREA D. GRABOVAC, MD
BRUNO A. CAYOUN, DPsych

New Harbinger Publications, Inc.

## Publisher's Note

*This publication is designed to provide accurate and authoritative information in regard to the subject matter covered. It is sold with the understanding that the publisher is not engaged in rendering psychological, financial, legal, or other professional services. If expert assistance or counseling is needed, the services of a competent professional should be sought.*

NEW HARBINGER PUBLICATIONS is a registered trademark of New Harbinger Publications, Inc.

New Harbinger Publications is an employee-owned company.

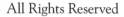

Copyright © 2024 by Andrea D. Grabovac and Bruno A. Cayoun

New Harbinger Publications, Inc.

5720 Shattuck Avenue

Oakland, CA 94609

www.newharbinger.com

All Rights Reserved

Cover design by Amy Daniel

Acquired by Wendy Millstine and Ryan Buresh

Edited by Max Sylvia

---

Library of Congress Cataloging-in-Publication Data on file

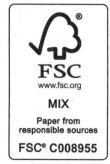

Printed in the United States of America

26    25    24

10    9    8    7    6    5    4    3    2    1                              First Printing

# Contents

# Introduction

"Laugh, and the world laughs with you; Weep, and you weep alone." Ella Wheeler Wilcox's words highlight the isolating sadness that can come with depression and anxiety (1883). This mindfulness-integrated cognitive behavior therapy (MiCBT) workbook is designed to equip you with evidence-based strategies to pave the way for more moments of shared joy and resilience in the face of life's challenges.

Our intention is not to eradicate discomfort; that would be an unrealistic pursuit. Instead, we aim to equip you with tools to encounter what life brings in a skillful manner. MiCBT is an evidence-based therapy which provides a structured pathway to transforming your relationship with anxiety and depression. It empowers you to cultivate a sense of agency and inner calm.

We've been privileged to work with thousands of individuals facing the challenges of anxiety and depression, drawing on decades of meditation practice and clinical experience in psychology and psychiatry in the process. Bruno has been a mindfulness meditator since 1989, practicing in the Burmese Vipassana tradition under S. N. Goenka, in the tradition of Ledi Sayadaw and U Ba Khin. Practices originating over twenty-five hundred years ago in northern India serve as the foundation for the techniques in this workbook.

For twelve years, Bruno harbored a dream—to forge a connection between clinical psychology and ancient mindfulness wisdom. He envisioned a world where the psychological insights derived from these timeless practices could be harnessed for the benefit of all. This unwavering aspiration propelled him to become a psychologist, setting the stage for the creation of MiCBT. On a parallel path for fifteen years before meeting Bruno, Andrea also practiced in a Burmese Vipassana tradition, dedicating her clinical and academic efforts to optimizing mindfulness training. Impressed by the structure and effectiveness of MiCBT, she partnered with Bruno, bringing her expertise to training other clinicians in this transformative method.

This book is secular in nature but draws upon tenets of Buddhist psychology and wisdom that have much to teach us about how we can navigate anxiety and depression, as well as the inevitable experiences of suffering that life brings. It includes an array of helpful exercises, reflections, and guided meditations to assist you in achieving improved well-being. In weeks 1 through 4, you'll learn to stabilize your thoughts and emotions to settle your mind. In weeks 5 and 6, you'll use these skills to reduce habits of avoidance and improve your confidence. During weeks 7 and 8, you'll apply mindfulness skills to the ways you communicate with people in tense situations. Finally, during weeks 9 and 10, you'll learn to abandon self-criticism and be kinder to yourself and others, in a way that helps prevent relapse into depression and anxiety.

We invite you to embark on this path of self-discovery, leveraging your current challenges with depression and anxiety as catalysts for change. As you dive in, recognize that the seeds of change are being sown. With patience and practice, they will flourish, leading to resilience and compassion. And we, drawing from our shared knowledge and experience, are here to guide, support, and encourage you every step of the way.

Welcome to a transformative journey toward healing and well-being.

# Part 1

# MiCBT Explained

## Chapter 1

# What Is MiCBT and How Can It Help Me?

Welcome to this empowering journey toward improving your well-being! In this chapter, we'll be exploring the four stages of the mindfulness-integrated cognitive behavior therapy program and the benefits of addressing depression and anxiety simultaneously. The MiCBT approach is *transdiagnostic*, meaning it also addresses other conditions, such as chronic pain, insomnia, or addictive behaviors, that often accompany and perpetuate depressive and anxiety symptoms. By applying the skills in this workbook to these conditions as well, you will significantly decrease the risk of falling back into old patterns and continue to cultivate your well-being going forward.

## Assessing Your Symptoms

Many, if not most, individuals who experience depression also experience anxiety. Decades of our own clinical experience and current research support the idea that anxiety and depression often go hand in hand.

When experiencing depression, feelings of dissatisfaction, lack of motivation, fatigue, and self-criticism can contribute to fear of remaining in this state of unhappiness. Over time, this fear or worry can lead to the development of anxiety symptoms. Research has shown that 85 percent of individuals with depression also experience symptoms of anxiety (Möller et al. 2016).

Similarly, anxiety symptoms such as constant worry, sleep struggles, and feeling restless, tense, and uncomfortable in the body can lead to feeling exhausted, unmotivated, and disheartened, leaving us with a sense of powerlessness or hopelessness. Prolonged anxiety symptoms can contribute to the development of depression.

Regardless of whether you first experience anxiety or depression, if one is present for an extended period, the other tends to develop, and symptoms become intertwined. This is not surprising given that there are similar brain changes in both conditions, and the same medications are often prescribed for both.

As you reflect on your own experience, have you noticed times when anxiety and depression were present at the same time? To further explore this connection, take a few minutes to mark the symptoms you have experienced in each of the three categories below: depression, anxiety, and symptoms common to both. This can be helpful in understanding the connection between the two conditions and how they may be affecting you.

| Depressive Symptoms | Anxiety Symptoms | Symptoms Found in Both Depression and Anxiety |
|---|---|---|
| ☐ Depressed/low mood | ☐ Feeling of impending danger/doom | ☐ Sleep disturbance (insomnia or oversleeping) |
| ☐ Sadness | ☐ Intrusive thoughts of danger | ☐ Restlessness (or agitation) |
| ☐ Loss of interest in usual activities | ☐ Hypervigilance | ☐ Fatigue |
| ☐ Loss of interest in pleasurable experiences | ☐ Fear of leaving one's home or being in crowded or open spaces | ☐ Irritability |
| ☐ Change in appetite | Physical symptoms of anxiety: | ☐ Excessive worrying |
| ☐ Sense of worthlessness | ☐ Rapid heart rate | ☐ Rumination (dwelling on negative thoughts and feelings) |
| ☐ Hopelessness | ☐ Irregular heartbeat | ☐ Difficulty concentrating |
| ☐ Feelings of guilt | ☐ Increased breathing rate | ☐ Difficulty with decision making |
| ☐ Loss of libido | ☐ Muscle tension | ☐ Social withdrawal |
| ☐ Thoughts of suicide or death | ☐ Sweating | Physical symptoms such as: |
| | ☐ Trembling | ☐ Headache |
| | ☐ Nausea | ☐ Stomachache |
| | | ☐ Chronic pain |

Seeing the individual symptoms of depression and anxiety written out can help us understand that while these conditions are difficult and painful to experience, they can also be seen as a collection of many individual experiences that are happening at the same time. It can take some practice, but when we see depression and anxiety in this way, we're less inclined to identify with each of the individual symptoms, and over time, we become less identified with the experience of depression and anxiety itself. This is because the whole appears to be greater than the sum of its parts, but once you see the parts, the whole is less overwhelming.

## How Can MiCBT Help?

MiCBT combines two important evidence-based therapeutic approaches: mindfulness training and cognitive behavior therapy (CBT). The mindfulness practices in MiCBT are designed to help you approach the symptoms of anxiety and depression objectively, and skillfully address any patterns of reactivity that may be maintaining them.

### Mindfulness

"Mindfulness" has become a bit of a buzzword these days, so it's important to clarify what we mean. Mindfulness is often defined as paying attention in the present moment without judgment, but it's also more than that. Informed by traditional Buddhist understanding, mindfulness can be described as a receptive, accepting, and nonreactive observation of our internal experience in the present moment (Grabovac, Lau, and Willett 2011). It is a way of relating to our inner experience without biased assumptions, reactivity, or identification with the experience. As we'll discuss in the next two chapters, *emotional reactivity* is the degree of intensity and swiftness with which one's emotions are triggered; it plays an important role in the development and maintenance of anxiety and depression.

Sometimes the description of mindfulness as a "nonjudgmental attitude" is misunderstood as needing to accept or agree with whatever is happening. On the contrary, mindfulness skills include carefully distinguishing between helpful and harmful actions, mental attitudes, and circumstances.

Mindfulness is not relaxation, although it can be very relaxing. It's not a way of changing how we feel in the moment or trying to feel calm or "better," although it can relieve distress. It's not about adopting a positive attitude or stopping our thoughts either, although it allows negative thoughts and attitudes to pass quickly.

In short, mindfulness is an unbiased tool for investigating the nature of our experience. As you embark on your journey with MiCBT, we invite you to use mindfulness skills to explore and understand your own experience, including how certain patterns in your thoughts, emotions, and behaviors can become associated with depression and anxiety. We'll explore these patterns objectively, in a way that's grounded in your direct experience. This can lead to valuable insights that support you in making informed and skillful choices to enhance your well-being.

## When Mindfulness Meets CBT

The integration of mindfulness and CBT in MiCBT offers many benefits, as these approaches complement each other in unique and powerful ways. CBT provides valuable skills for changing the *content* of unhelpful beliefs, while mindfulness offers a practical and effective approach to understanding and changing the *processes* or *mechanisms* of our thinking. Additionally, mindfulness helps us recognize early signs of emotions in the body and prevent reactivity, while CBT teaches strategies for changing our unhelpful behaviors once we recognize what's driving them. Lastly, CBT also provides a systematic way of applying mindfulness skills in daily life.

The sophisticated integration of core CBT skills with mindfulness training in MiCBT does not allow any aspect of thoughts, emotions, or behaviors to fall through the cracks, so to speak. All aspects of anxiety and depression can be addressed.

# The MiCBT Program

In this section, we provide a brief outline of the structure and content of the MiCBT program, which has four stages, each focusing on different aspects of your well-being.

## Stage 1

Stage 1, the personal stage of MiCBT, focuses on skills that address internal experiences such as unhelpful thoughts and emotions. During this stage, presented in weeks 1 to 4 of the MiCBT program, you'll begin by gently training your mind to stay in the present moment, using your body as an anchor for attention during progressive muscle relaxation practice. The more you're able to focus on the present, the less likely you are to be worrying about the future or ruminating about the past. You will also learn to relax any potential muscle tension through this practice. This will not only help you recognize the difference between tension and relaxation during daily life but can also be a rewarding method of self-care.

The following week, you'll learn how to not engage in ruminative, obsessive, and catastrophic thinking by training awareness of thoughts during the practice of mindfulness of breath. In the last two weeks of stage 1, body scanning practices are introduced. These train the ability to feel physical sensations with acceptance and nonreactivity, and through this process you'll begin to decrease distressing emotions. Over the course of stage 1, you'll develop the ability to regulate attention and emotion and to significantly reduce your symptoms.

## Stage 2

Stage 2, the exposure stage, is designed to help you work with and overcome avoidance of situations, as avoidance maintains anxiety and depressive symptoms. You'll practice two mindfulness-based exposure methods, one using imagery and the other using real-life situations. Stage 2 typically takes about two weeks to complete (weeks 5 and 6 of the program). During this time, you'll become more confident and able to readily approach situations and contexts you might once have avoided.

## Stage 3

In stage 3, or the interpersonal stage, presented in weeks 7 and 8, you develop skills that help reduce your fear of conflict and improve your ability to express your views and needs more effectively. By applying specific mindfulness skills in challenging interactions, you can learn to remain empathic while communicating clearly and confidently. This helps you set stronger personal boundaries and can lead to improved relationships.

## Stage 4

Stage 4, or weeks 9 and 10, is called the "compassion stage" because we focus on cultivating compassion grounded in kind and ethical actions towards ourselves and others. This helps prevent relapse into depression and anxiety by fostering a deeper sense of connection with others. During this stage and in the daily maintenance practice that follows, we prioritize developing ten skills and attitudes to support you in aligning your actions with your values, both in small day-to-day decisions and in larger life choices. Stage 4 can feel like the culmination of a transformative journey and the beginning of a new chapter of life, filled with possibilities and opportunities.

## Committing to Learning and Changing

The effectiveness of the MiCBT approach depends on your commitment to practicing the skills it teaches. We understand that change can be challenging. It's also completely normal to have moments of doubt or uncertainty when it comes to change, especially regarding mental health. That's why, as we begin this journey together, it is important to take a moment to reflect on your readiness for change.

A mindful stance toward our lives includes the ability to recognize both what we can't change and what we can. It is common to find yourself feeling that aspects of the situation you're in need to change before *you* can change. People who attend therapy sessions often say, "I wish my husband were different," or "I wish my sister could change." Parents might say, "I want my child to be more respectful," while their teenagers say, "My parents don't understand me at all." We can ask ourselves whether we're ready to take responsibility for addressing the situation we find ourselves in, and accept that we may need to make some changes to the ways we respond, even if our control over the situations themselves is limited.

Are you willing to put in consistent effort and dedication to achieve your goals? If you commit to practicing the skills, you can experience real change in just a matter of weeks.

To achieve the change you desire, let's start by identifying the specific things you would like to change. These are your *targeted problems*. Next, to help you measure the effectiveness of your progress, you'll need clear *success indicators* for each targeted problem.

## Choosing Targeted Problems

When setting your goals for change, it's important to focus on what you can control and influence. When selecting up to five targeted problems, choose the most obvious ones. Don't worry if there are things you want to change that aren't addressed by the specific issues you choose now; the skills you learn in this program can be applied to other concerns in the future. For now, we want to narrow our scope to a few areas that feel both manageable and useful. Common targeted problems include difficulty falling asleep, loneliness, not getting enough exercise, setting boundaries in relationships, low motivation, rumination, panic attacks, anger, and social anxiety.

Note that while some of these targeted problems may involve other people's behavior, it's important to focus on how you experience and respond to that behavior. For example, instead of writing "My teenage son acts disrespectfully towards me," in the table below, reframe the targeted problem to focus on your experience—"Feeling helpless and powerless when my son acts disrespectfully"—because *your* experience and behavior are things that *you* can change. Examples of targeted problems can be found in the next table.

## Identifying Success Indicators

For each targeted problem, identify two or three success indicators. These should be specific, measurable goals that will help you track your progress. The more detailed and behaviorally based your success indicators are, the easier it will be to tell whether you have successfully met your goals.

Using the example of "difficulty falling asleep," instead of a vague goal like "Sleeping better," three specific success indicators could be: "Falling asleep within 30 minutes of going to bed," "Not ruminating in bed," and "Implementing my bedtime routine six nights a week." In the example of feeling helpless when your child acts disrespectfully, specific success indicators could be: "Have a conversation about our communication without me reacting angrily," "Ask him about his perspective on a situation several times a week," and "Listen without interrupting."

See below for more examples of useful success indicators. Then, use the table that follows to list at least three target problems and identify up to three success indicators for each problem.

| Targeted Problems | Success Indicators |
|---|---|
| 1. Feeling worthless | A. Tidying my living space for 30 minutes 4 times a week as a way of valuing myself |
| | B. Exercising 4 days a week |
| | C. Prioritizing my health by eating one nutritious snack daily |
| 2. Ruminating over being unemployed | A. Redirecting my thoughts to a more constructive topic within 3 minutes |
| | B. Dedicating at least 30 minutes 4 days a week to actively search for job opportunities |
| | C. Submitting 3 job applications a week |
| 3. Feeling lonely and socially isolated | A. Volunteering 2 hours each week |
| | B. Arranging to go for coffee with a friend at least once a week |
| | C. Joining the local walking club and walking at least twice weekly |

| Targeted Problems | Success Indicators |
|---|---|
| | |
| | |
| | |
| | |
| | |
| | |
| | |
| | |
| | |

Now that you've identified specific changes you'd like to make, we'll look at how you'll get there.

If you can, close your eyes and allow yourself to genuinely imagine what life would be like for you if you achieved all these success indicators. Then imagine what it would be like for people you care for. These goals are attainable with one core component of MiCBT: the consistent practice of mindfulness.

## Regular Practice of Mindfulness Meditation

Whereas reading *informs* you, practice *transforms* you. The purpose of MiCBT is to transform the thoughts and behaviors underlying the experience of depression and anxiety. Daily meditation practice transforms you because it changes how various parts of the brain process information, from ways that maintain symptoms of depression and anxiety to ways that support resilience and well-being. As you may have noticed while reflecting on your symptoms, much of depression and anxiety has to do with particular patterns of thinking and feeling that influence behavior. When we think worrying thoughts or ruminate on things out of our control, or feel restless, guilty, hopeless, irritable, or sad, it's likely that it is difficult to concentrate, relax, or sleep. Mindfulness allows you to understand how these patterns of thinking, feeling, and behaving stem from the ways our brains perceive and interpret experience.

While reading can be very helpful for understanding how mindfulness works to treat depression and anxiety, or how to practice mindfulness effectively, it is the daily practice of mindfulness skills that actually changes neural connections in the brain in ways that make it possible to intervene in anxiety and depression. We'll discuss this in more detail in chapter 3.

For any skills-training approach, there are three key components to successful learning. These are:

- Sufficient *frequency* of practice: how often we train the skills

- Sufficient *duration* of practice: how long each practice session lasts

- Sufficient *accuracy* of practice: how precisely we practice the skills

To obtain the results typically achieved with MiCBT, it's essential to adhere to these three conditions. We recommend practicing mindfulness meditation twice daily, for 30 minutes per session, and with a focus on accuracy as outlined in this workbook and accompanying audio instructions, which can be found at http://www.newharbinger.com/52571.

This might sound like an intensive commitment, but consider: would committing to a consistent practice of mindfulness meditation for ten weeks be a worthwhile investment if doing so could bring relief from depression and anxiety?

# What MiCBT Makes Possible

By using the mindfulness tools and other techniques outlined in this book, you'll develop a deeper understanding of five key skills that are trained in MiCBT:

1.  Attention regulation: training to regain control over your mind

2.  Emotional regulation: decreasing reactivity

3.  Behavioral regulation: reducing avoidant behaviors

4.  Interpersonal regulation: communicating mindfully and confidently

5.  Transpersonal regulation: decreasing potential for relapse through compassion for self and others

We'll explore both the reasons and the steps for developing these five skills, which will work together to decrease your symptoms and improve your well-being. We'll also closely examine the cultivation of equanimity—the objective, nonreactive attitude toward your internal experience—that is the foundation for these skills.

By committing to practicing mindfulness meditation twice daily and completing the other exercises outlined in this book, you'll develop a deeper awareness of the relationship between thoughts and body sensations. You'll also learn the skills needed to reduce the hold that anxiety and depression can have on your life, opening space for improved relationships that truly meet your needs and the experience of genuine compassion and care for yourself and those around you.

## Some Precautions

There are a few potential contraindications for using MiCBT and other mindfulness-based therapies to be aware of before you move forward. MiCBT should not be used if you're experiencing active symptoms of mania or psychosis.

Also, remember that everyone's journey is different. If you are struggling with severe anxiety or depression, or if you have other complex issues such as a history of trauma or addiction, it may be helpful to work with a therapist—ideally one trained in MiCBT. If you do decide to work with a therapist, keep in mind that not all mindfulness-based therapies are the same. Some methods may not align with the approach outlined in this book, so make sure that your therapist is comfortable working with you using these specific techniques.

## Change Agreement

We invite you to join us on this journey of self-discovery and growth, and to make this commitment to yourself by signing and dating the Change Agreement below.

---

### Change Agreement

I have identified specific targeted problems, established clear success indicators, and have written these out in the table above.

I commit to practicing mindfulness meditation twice daily and completing the other exercises outlined in this workbook.

_____          _____

Signature                                                                      Date

---

Remember that progress and growth don't happen in a straight line; be kind and compassionate to yourself throughout this process.

## Chapter 2

# What Causes and Maintains Unhappiness?

*Suffering* encompasses any experience causing dissatisfaction or emotional reactivity, ranging from subtle to devastating events. While it can seem that external factors, such as losses or financial difficulties, are the cause of unhappiness, it is often our underlying expectations for what "should" or "shouldn't" be happening that most influence how we feel. Though suffering can feel isolating, it is a universal experience. We all encounter unfulfilled hopes and daily challenges. We may get temporary relief through avoidance or wishing things were different, but trying to escape suffering can ultimately intensify our discomfort and contribute to feeling anxious or depressed.

In this chapter, we'll look at how suffering is conceptualized in Buddhist psychology. As you'll discover, it is an approach that acknowledges the reality of suffering and illuminates how the ways we instinctively respond to suffering can inadvertently prolong it. You'll also begin to explore how the causes of suffering—craving, aversion, and unawareness—may be manifesting in your own life, in preparation for the work you'll do in part 2. Let's begin.

## The Three Types of Suffering

We may question whether suffering itself causes anxiety or depression, or if it is anxiety and depression that lead to suffering. Understanding the causes of suffering and related unhappiness can be complex, and it is important to approach this exploration with curiosity and openness. We can gain insight into this dynamic through careful observation. MiCBT, informed by the teachings of Buddhist psychology (Bodhi 2005), offers a practical framework for understanding how unhappiness is created in our lives.

Let's take a look at the three main types of suffering, in order to further explore their causes.

| Suffering Related to Conditioning | Suffering Related to Illness and Injury | Suffering Related to Change |
|---|---|---|

## Suffering Related to Conditioning

Suffering is often acquired through learning, or *conditioning*, which occurs in three main ways. The first, *social conditioning*, involves learning from observing others. The second, *operant conditioning*, involves learning from the consequences of our actions, like using alcohol to temporarily reduce anxiety. The third, *classical conditioning*, refers to learning through associations, such as associating a specific location with having a panic attack. These learning methods can either maintain our suffering or help us establish more helpful patterns.

Our sense of who we are is also the result of a continual learning process, and our perception of happiness and unhappiness relies heavily on our learned sense of self-worth. Those of us with low self-worth may blame ourselves, and think, *I'm not good enough*, while some may blame others for their unhappiness, and think, *It's their fault I feel this way*.

Reflect on how you typically understand and attribute your experiences of suffering. Are you inclined toward one end of the spectrum or are you more in the middle? Answer the following questions honestly and without judgment, as understanding our tendencies allows us to challenge our perspectives and develop a more compassionate understanding of ourselves and others.

What are some habitual thoughts or behaviors you've developed that might be contributing to your anxious thoughts or depressed feelings?

_____

_____

_____

_____

_____

_____

_____

What ideas do you have about how they are being reinforced? How might conditioning, based on your life circumstances, be playing a role in instigating or perpetuating them?

_____

_____

_____

_____

## Suffering Related to Illness or Injury

So many things are unpredictable in our lives. One thing we can all be sure of is that, at some point, we or someone we care for will experience an injury or illness. This can be one of the most difficult things we face in life. When this happens, it's natural to have thoughts like *Why me?* or *It's not fair that this is happening to them!* Our attachment to our bodies and loved ones can make us feel anxious and aggrieved.

The Buddha's teachings on the "two arrows" can help us understand the nature of this kind of suffering and how to approach it in a truly accurate and compassionate way. Imagine you are walking in the woods and suddenly an arrow strikes your arm, causing intense pain. This "first arrow" represents the situation that's causing you pain, such as the experiences of acute injury or chronic illness. Situations like these are an inevitable part of human experience. When we are shot by this first arrow, our mind can start to question what's happening—*What did I do to deserve this?*—or race with thoughts of worst-case scenarios, such as *What if I never get better?* The "second arrow" represents the suffering we create for ourselves through our judgement and emotional reactivity to the pain caused by the first arrow. The pain of the first arrow is unavoidable, but we can learn to not shoot the second arrow.

Have you, or people you care for, experienced physical illness or injury? If so, write some examples here.

_____

_____

_____

_____

Did you find yourself reacting with catastrophic thoughts that negatively impacted your mood, caused anxiety, or made it difficult to move forward? If so, jot down some alternative thoughts that might have been less distressing.

_____

_____

_____

_____

_____

## Suffering Related to Change

Life's ever-changing nature reminds us that nothing is permanent. You may have noticed that the things we want seem to happen only occasionally, while the things we don't want seem to occur often. And when we get what we want, it eventually changes—and if it doesn't, _we_ do! Still, we often strive to achieve an imagined ideal state, believing happiness and contentment will follow. We pursue grander homes, avoid challenges, or seek new relationships, only to encounter dissatisfaction when circumstances inevitably change. This sense of dissatisfaction can be very subtle, yet pervasive. By cultivating the awareness that changes are a natural, inescapable part of life, we can navigate them more skillfully.

Reflect on a time in your life when you were feeling a sense of peace or contentment. When circumstances changed, how did you feel?

_____

_____

_____

_____

_____

Reflect on this experience of change. How did you meet it at the time? Perhaps with acceptance and allowing, or perhaps with resistance and resentment? Jot down any tendencies or common patterns you recognize in yourself when unwanted change occurs.

_____

_____

_____

_____

_____

_____

Fundamentally, what connects these three types of suffering—suffering related to the ways we've been conditioned; to illness, injury, and pain; and to the inevitable changes we encounter—is that they all have three underlying causes: craving, aversion, and unawareness. Understanding these causes can help us recognize them in our own lives and take effective steps towards reducing our suffering.

## The Three Universal Causes of Suffering

Suffering, according to Buddhist psychology, springs from three fundamental causes: craving for pleasant experiences we cannot have, aversion to unpleasant experiences we do have and don't want, and a lack of awareness of the impermanence of all things, including our very sense of self. Buddhist psychology and MiCBT outline how we can work constructively with each of these causes of suffering to mitigate its effects.

| Craving | Aversion | Unawareness |

## Craving

Craving is the impulse to obtain pleasant sensations, such as the taste of good food, the profound fulfillment of a pleasurable sexual experience, or the kind of life we used to have. Craving arises as the consequence of past attachments. Dissatisfaction occurs because we crave these kinds of pleasurable sensations when they are not available to us. We often believe they will bring us lasting happiness and satisfaction, but in reality all experiences are temporary. No matter how much we enjoy them, they will eventually end, leaving us with the same sense of dissatisfaction—unless we can come to accept their ephemerality.

To work skillfully with craving, we can develop *equanimity*, a balanced state in which we can fully enjoy pleasurable experiences without feeling empty or dissatisfied when they inevitably change or end. We'll explore equanimity in greater detail in the next chapter and begin developing it in week 3.

## Aversion

Aversion is the impulse to avoid or resist something we dislike, whether it is an external experience or something occurring within our body or mind. It is based on the idea that we can effectively avoid, escape, or push away feelings of unpleasantness, which is ultimately an illusion. Like craving, aversion is conditioned and arises from previous disliked experiences.

Aversion is often maintained or increased by our beliefs and assumptions about the world. We may believe that we have significant control over our experiences and can dictate outcomes. Although we do indeed have some control over our circumstances, there will always be parts of life that escape our influence. We may feel frustrated, angry, or hopeless when things don't unfold as we want them to.

To illustrate aversion further, consider the case of someone who has experienced trauma, such as a car accident. They may develop a strong aversion to driving. This avoidance is understandable; it provides some relief from the unpleasant sensations of anxiety and fear. But it can also have a negative impact on their daily life. They may have difficulty getting to work or running errands, and their social life may be affected. The longer they allow aversion toward the discomfort associated with driving to dictate the choices they make, the more entrenched that fear becomes.

*Mindfulness-based exposure*—the practice of gradually encountering the sensations associated with anxiety and fear, in a safe way, with equanimity, rather than trying to avoid or suppress them—can be helpful in addressing this type of aversion. We will be learning this set of skills in weeks 5 and 6.

## Unawareness

Unawareness as a universal cause of suffering emerges from an entrenched misunderstanding of the transient nature of reality—that all things change continually. This includes our very sense of identity, what we consider "I" or "me."

Often, in the throes of anxiety or depression, we might think things like *I really want to feel less anxious, but I'm a worrier; that's just who I am.* We can start to identify with our thoughts and emotions and believe they represent who we are. But the reality is life is constantly changing. This includes our thoughts, feelings, sensations, and even our sense of self, what we call "I" or "me." Recognizing this reality, which has been called "the law of impermanence" (Hart 1987), can help us understand that everything is transitory—including our self-concepts in a given moment, no matter how compelling, true, or "sticky" they might seem.

What are some of the self-concepts that you struggle with? For example, "I am not likeable," or "I am not good at learning new skills." If we were to ask you to complete the sentence, "I am…," what negative descriptions would come up for you?

_____

_____

_____

_____

_____

Accepting the law of impermanence can be challenging, especially when we're taught to believe that we have fixed traits or identities.

In addition, we're often encouraged to hold on to experiences we enjoy and avoid ones we don't like. But it's also true, as you've no doubt experienced, that no attempt to control what we experience is 100 percent effective, 100 percent of the time. We may try to avoid an unpleasant moment, a painful sensation, or a destructive thought, and sometimes we might succeed, but odds are that similar moments, sensations, and thoughts will arise again despite our best efforts to prevent them. By embracing impermanence, we move away from struggling with what we can't control, toward engaging with the fluidity of our identities, life's varying joys and pains, and the transient nature of all experiences.

# Changing from Within

Depression and anxiety are often accompanied by a feeling of inadequacy or dissatisfaction with ourselves. We may feel that we're not good enough or that we're not living up to our potential. As long as we continue to cling to the belief that we'll be happy once things are a certain way, we are setting ourselves up for disappointment. We will never be able to fulfill all our expectations and desires in this way.

Meet one of our patients, whom we will call Susan. She has two young adult children who have recently left home. She had been working hard towards her goal of reaching the senior level at the non-profit she worked for and enjoyed her job. However, issues of chronic pain stymied her to a degree, and during a difficult divorce from her partner, she developed depression and was unable to continue working. She felt embarrassed about her struggles and found herself declining her friends' invitations to spend time together; it felt easier to just avoid everyone. But she longed for the way things used to be: having a fulfilling job and a good social life and living pain-free.

Despite her troubles, Susan was able to seek help from her doctor and started an antidepressant and new pain medication. After about three weeks, she noticed an improvement in her symptoms. She reconnected with several of her friends and even met someone new. But this happiness proved to be short-lived. Her new partner, Rob, ended their relationship due to unresolved issues with his ex-wife. And some of Susan's friends were often unavailable due to family obligations. Feeling rejected and worthless, Susan took the situation personally and ended up isolating herself once again. Ultimately, Susan had a hard time accepting that circumstances are constantly changing, in ways both pleasant and unpleasant—and that her previous life was likely not coming back.

In this period of Susan's life, the trigger or precipitating factor for her dissatisfaction was *change* in her relationship and health, leading to divorce, depression, and job loss. She experienced ongoing *aversion* to her situation and *craving* for the future to be like her past; she wanted her previous life back. She was *unaware*, or perhaps unwilling to recognize, that situations keep changing, at times in unwanted directions. The same cycle of suffering repeated itself when her new partner was no longer available, and when she craved the company of her friends. Her dislike of who she believed she was also increased, and she identified as being worthless and a failure. Her doctor then referred her for treatment with MiCBT.

Susan's story is unfortunately common. If you look carefully, you may notice that you too have a tendency to identify with your experiences, despite their impermanence. This is a fundamental subconscious mechanism that reinforces unhappiness for many of us. The table below has examples of how craving, aversion, and unawareness of impermanence can affect our thoughts and behaviors when we feel depressed or anxious.

| Cause of Suffering | Examples of Anxious Thoughts | Examples of Depressive Thoughts |
|---|---|---|
| **Craving**<br><br>The impulse to satisfy a desire; an unfulfilled expectation or desire for something to be different than it is | • I can't help it; I overeat to reduce my anxiety.<br>• I'm so worried I won't get the promotion that I can't sleep. | • I need to have someone at home with me all the time; otherwise, I'll feel empty.<br>• What's the point of getting out of bed if I don't have the money I need to pay my bills? |
| **Aversion**<br><br>The avoidance of, or resistance toward, something we dislike, whether external to us or occurring in our body or mind | • I don't like flying because I can't handle the anxiety when the plane takes off.<br>• I'm not leaving the house today because I don't want to have a panic attack in public.<br>• I'm afraid of going to bed at night in case I have another nightmare. | • I hate myself.<br>• There's no point in looking for a job because I'm not good at anything.<br>• All the bad things that have happened to my children since the divorce are my fault. |
| **Unawareness of Impermanence**<br><br>Not recognizing that everything is temporary, including our moment-to-moment internal experiences | • What if I continue to feel anxious all my life?<br>• If I stop overworking, I'll lose my position in the department and will never have another chance.<br>• What if I fall and permanently injure myself? | • I'm just like my father; I'll never change.<br>• We were so happy together before we had kids.<br>• I hate my body. I want to be attractive like I was ten years ago. |

Again, the core insight here is that our thoughts, emotions, and experiences are fleeting and constantly changing. No matter how much we become attached to the pleasant ones, they will eventually change. How can we be satisfied if we're always clinging to experiences that are bound to change? And though we may try to avoid unpleasant experiences, they will inevitably occur.

Can you think of examples in your own life when you experienced disappointment because you craved something that was no longer available? If so, write them here.

_____

_____

_____

_____

_____

_____

Considering your present day-to-day experiences, are there situations or circumstances that you try to avoid because they are difficult or unpleasant? List some of them here.

_____

_____

_____

_____

_____

_____

If you were to "soften" or identify less strongly with beliefs about who you are or thoughts you have, how might that make a difference for you?

_____

_____

_____

_____

_____

_____

Are there challenges to identifying less strongly with beliefs about who you are? Do you find resistance coming up? Take a moment to acknowledge these experiences before you read on.

_____

_____

_____

_____

_____

_____

_____

_____

_____

It's not always easy. But by letting go of your attachment to things being a certain way—including your beliefs about who you are, or about how life must be—you can allow yourself to change when change is needed and begin to move towards a more accepting and compassionate way of living. This can help you see yourself and others differently and more clearly. It can also lead you to a greater sense of well-being and happiness.

## Moving Forward

Depression and anxiety, although distinct, share the same underlying causes: craving, aversion, and a lack of awareness of impermanence. These mechanisms influence our emotional processing and contribute to suffering. However, they can be tempered and transformed through mindfulness training like MiCBT. In the following chapter, we will explore how this can be effectively achieved through the "co-emergence model of reinforcement" (Cayoun and Shires 2020).

## Chapter 3

# Creating a Flexible and Resilient Inner Equilibrium

In this chapter, we delve into the co-emergence model of reinforcement, the foundation of the MiCBT approach to working skillfully with emotional reactivity. Understanding this mechanism of change will deepen your knowledge and enhance the effectiveness of the practices taught in MiCBT. It will show you how the suffering of depression and anxiety can be addressed by restoring equilibrium in the way we think, feel, and respond to life stresses. Coupled with *neuroplasticity*, the adaptive changes in the brain induced by mindfulness practice, this knowledge can help you break free from unhelpful habits and develop healthier thought patterns and behaviors.

## The Co-Emergence Model of Reinforcement

The *co-emergence model of reinforcement* (Cayoun and Shires 2020) combines a neuroscience-based understanding of emotions and behavior with Buddhist psychology to explain how we learn to react or respond in certain ways. It is based on a particular way of understanding our experience known as embodied cognition (Varela et al. 1991). *Embodied cognition* posits that the mind and body cannot be separated—our mental functions and bodily experiences are intertwined.

The diagram on the next page illustrates the five components of the co-emergence model of reinforcement. Together, the components of the model describe how our mind and body are interconnected and influence each other to produce behavior.

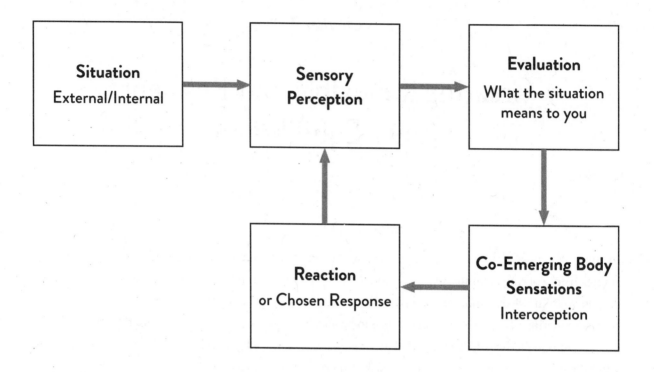

## Situation

This first component, situation, represents the stimulus or context for experiences we have. It can be external to us, such as getting honked at by a nearby car, or passed over for a promotion, or it can be internal, such as physical pain, a pleasant sense of fullness after a meal, or mental activity, such as thoughts or images.

## Sensory Perception

Sensory perception, the second component, represents our ability to perceive sensory information through our five physical senses—smell, sight, taste, touch, and hearing—as well as our ability to feel internal body sensations, which is called *interoception* or *interoceptive awareness*, and our perception of our thoughts as they enter our consciousness, which is called *metacognition*. These "seven senses" allow us to experience the world around and within us. This is how we know that a situation (the first component) is taking place.

## Evaluation

The process of evaluation, represented by the third box in the model, is a unique and personal experience for each individual. As incoming sensory information is filtered and processed, we make sense of the situation based on our personal frame of reference. This frame of reference is shaped by our past experiences, and includes our beliefs, values, cultural influences, needs, moods, and preferences, all of which act as filters and influence our decisions and actions.

This efficient system has evolved over thousands of years for survival purposes, allowing us to quickly and effectively assess if a situation is safe or poses a threat. Our minds are naturally wired to make these quick and effective judgments and decisions through the use of belief systems known as *schemas*. Our schemas encompass both conscious beliefs and deeper, fundamental core beliefs that shape our everyday assumptions and perceptions, often going unnoticed since childhood.

While the automaticity of schemas can be beneficial in certain situations, they can also lead to inaccurate assessments and false alarms, as not all beliefs are necessarily factual or helpful. Some examples of maladaptive beliefs include: *I need to do everything myself to ensure it's done right*, *Committed relationships are not worth the effort because people can't be trusted*, and *It's better to stay with someone who is abusive than to be alone*. These kinds of beliefs can lead to unpleasant sensations in the body, destructive emotions, and unhelpful behavior.

Adaptive schemas, on the other hand, support us in approaching difficult situations more skillfully, as they are associated with helpful thoughts and beliefs. Typical examples are *I have the skills to figure this out*, *While I'm not perfect, I am lovable*, and *Nobody is coming to speak to me at this party, but that's probably because I haven't said hello to anyone yet*. When adaptive beliefs are activated, they are either not accompanied by intense sensations in the body or result in the co-emergence of pleasant ones and associated helpful behaviors.

In summary, evaluation represents what the situations we encounter mean to us. For example, we may have the thought, *I forgot to call my brother on his birthday*, and the resulting conscious belief may be, *He'll be upset with me*. At a deeper and perhaps preconscious level, the unhelpful core belief may be *I'm a disappointment to others; I can't get anything right*, stemming from an underlying schema of worthlessness.

## Co-Emerging Body Sensations

This natural, automatic process of evaluating the situations we encounter affects the body immediately. When you have thoughts about matters that are important to you, they are accompanied by sensations that emerge at the same time in your body, hence the term "co-emergence." These could include tension when you're stressed, lightness when you're joyful, heaviness when you're sad, constriction in the chest or "butterflies" in your stomach when you're anxious. These are represented by the fourth component of the model.

Co-emerging sensations are experienced through interoception. These body sensations are described as "co-emerging" specifically because they emerge simultaneously with our evaluative thoughts. It may not always seem this way, but these sensations are the direct consequences of our *thoughts* about a situation, not the situation itself—and it is helpful to keep this in mind.

You may also have noticed that the kinds of thoughts you have affect how the co-emerging sensations feel in the body. If we believe a situation is positive for ourselves, those we care about, or for society or the environment, we will likely experience pleasant sensations in the body. On the other hand, if we believe a situation is negative, we will likely experience unpleasant sensations. In other words, our schemas and accompanying evaluations determine the type or qualities of the body sensations, with pleasant thoughts resulting in pleasant sensations, and unpleasant thoughts resulting in unpleasant sensations.

For example, during a period of depression, have you ever had a morning where you woke up feeling drained and overwhelmed, with thoughts like *What's the point of getting up? I'll just stay in bed today.* If you have, you may have noticed that these thoughts were accompanied by unpleasant sensations in your body. These sensations may have felt like heaviness in certain areas, amplifying feelings of fatigue, or a hollowness or sinking feeling in your stomach. At other times, you may have experienced anxious thoughts about an event later in the day, and these would have co-emerged with unpleasant sensations, even if you weren't consciously aware of them at the time. These may have included tightness in the chest, stomach, or neck, and possibly an agitated feeling in your body in the form of increased heart rate, trembling, or tingling sensations.

Of course, if you have depression and anxiety, it can be normal to not be very aware of your bodily sensations at all. Still, the next time depressed or anxious thoughts arise, you might try to attend to the sensations that co-emerge in your body, to begin to observe the co-emergence process as it operates.

Interestingly, the intensity and type of co-emerging sensations can also be influenced by our memories, or even by past experiences that we can no longer specifically recall. Sometimes, even the simplest things like seeing someone's face or hearing their voice can immediately evoke pleasant or unpleasant sensations in our body, depending on how underlying schemas affect our interpretation of the situation. Suppose someone reminds you, even subconsciously, of a person you liked or loved in the past. In that case, the co-emerging sensations might be pleasant, and you might feel compelled to prolong your time with them. On the other hand, if the co-emerging sensations are unpleasant, you might naturally try to avoid further reminders. Behaviorally, this shows up as craving or aversion, as introduced in the previous chapter.

The intensity and type of co-emerging sensations can also be influenced by the degree of personal relevance and identification with the situation. The more our evaluations are related to ourselves or to something or someone we value, the stronger the sensations that will co-emerge!

Why does all this matter? Because by becoming more aware of these body sensations, we can learn to use them as a source of information about our emotional state and the situations we are facing. We also become more able to take responsibility for what we feel before reacting. This ability is critical to interrupting the cycle that anxious and depressive thoughts and any related co-emerging sensations can lock us into.

## Experiencing the Effects of Context on Co-Emerging Body Sensations

The following exercise will support you in exploring the effects of context on thoughts and their co-emerging sensations. You can choose to close your eyes as you visualize each scenario, as this can help you feel body sensations in more detail during the visualization. Some of the scenarios you'll be asked to envision may feel intense; take the time you need while you do this visualization.

### Scenario 1

Imagine that you are listening to a radio announcement about a person you don't know who was in a car accident 250 miles away from you and was hospitalized. Take a moment to visualize the scene—where you are standing or sitting, the voice of the radio broadcaster, etc.

*On a scale of 0 to 10, rate the intensity of any co-emerging sensations you feel while imagining this scenario. A 0 means you don't feel any sensations, and a 10 means you feel the co-emerging sensations intensely.*

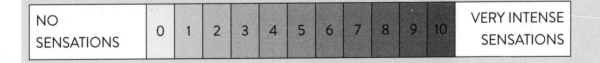

| NO SENSATIONS | 0 | 1 | 2 | 3 | 4 | 5 | 6 | 7 | 8 | 9 | 10 | VERY INTENSE SENSATIONS |
|---|---|---|---|---|---|---|---|---|---|---|---|---|

### Scenario 2

Now, imagine the same radio announcement, but this time the person involved in the accident is a very good friend of yours. Are there any co-emerging sensations in your body?

On a scale of 0 to 10, rate the intensity of any co-emerging sensations you feel while imagining this scenario.

| NO SENSATIONS | 0 | 1 | 2 | 3 | 4 | 5 | 6 | 7 | 8 | 9 | 10 | VERY INTENSE SENSATIONS |
|---|---|---|---|---|---|---|---|---|---|---|---|---|

## Scenario 3

Finally, if it feels manageable, imagine the same radio announcement, but this time it's about someone close to you that you care about deeply, such as a partner, child, or parent.

On a scale of 0 to 10, rate the intensity of any co-emerging sensations you feel while imagining this scenario.

| NO SENSATIONS | 0 | 1 | 2 | 3 | 4 | 5 | 6 | 7 | 8 | 9 | 10 | VERY INTENSE SENSATIONS |
|---|---|---|---|---|---|---|---|---|---|---|---|---|

If you noticed a difference in the intensity of the co-emerging sensations between these three scenarios, you have just experienced how the degree to which we identify with a situation influences the sensations we feel. Often, the extent to which a thought is related to "I," "me," and "mine" determines the intensity of the co-emerging sensations.

## Reaction or Response

The fifth component of the co-emergence model, reaction or response, is our reaction or response to the co-emerging sensations we are experiencing. If the sensations are pleasant, in addition to liking them, we are likely to react with a desire to experience more of them. Becoming attached to sensations will lead to craving them during times when we cannot have them. Can you recognize one of the causes of suffering here?

Similarly, suppose the co-emerging sensations are unpleasant. In addition to disliking them, we are likely to react with a desire to have less of them (i.e., to avoid them). Later, we are more likely to feel aversion and resent them when they arise again.

Our biological system has evolved to promote behaviors that increase pleasant sensations and decrease unpleasant ones. This kept our ancestors safe. The sweet, pleasant-tasting berries were safe to eat and were sought out. The bitter, unpleasant ones were poisonous and to be avoided! It is very understandable, then, that our neurobiology is wired in such a way.

Suppose we are successful at decreasing unpleasant sensations. In that case, the behavior through which we accomplished this will be reinforced by the accompanying sense of relief and, therefore, more likely to happen again. Say the thought of speaking up in front of your coworkers at an important meeting drives your anxiety up, leaving your palms sweaty and your heart racing. You might think, *I can't possibly do that!* You might choose to call in sick the night before to avoid the situation, or not say anything during the meeting. And you would probably feel some immediate relief from not needing to face that responsibility anymore. Odds are that sense of relief would then reinforce your avoidance of feeling anxious, making you more predisposed to avoid the experience of anxiety again next time it spikes.

As may be clear by now, avoiding your anxiety in this way leaves the anxiety itself unchallenged. You might also find fearful or depressive thoughts coming up, like *Will there be consequences for missing that meeting? I can't believe I had to make an excuse,* or *Will I ever get over this?* In this way, our reactions to body sensations co-emerging with the prospect of public speaking, accompanied by the thought *I can't possibly do that,* can perpetuate the cycle of anxiety and depression.

In the next section, we look at what these five boxes look like when the experience of depression and anxiety becomes a persistent part of our daily life.

## Anxiety and Depression as Consequences of Disequilibrium

When life's stressors persist or occur frequently, it can feel like we've lost our sense of balance. Overthinking, overreacting, being less objective, and feeling emotionally disconnected may start to feel like our usual way of being. When this occurs, the way we process information is in a *disequilibrium state*.

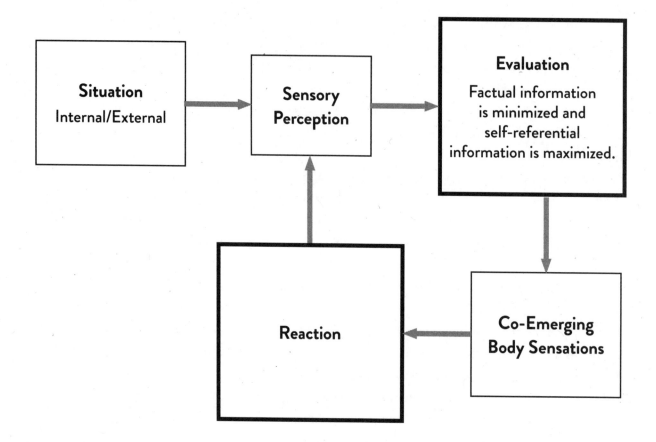

When information processing is in disequilibrium, we're less able to pay attention to objective information coming through our five senses and body sensations—represented in the diagram by a reduction in size of the Sensory Perception box—and we automatically rely more on past experiences stored in memory to make sense of the situation. This is especially the case when a situation is ambiguous and we cannot predict the outcome. In fact, the brain has evolved to constantly be making predictions about our environment and the potential consequences of our future behaviors—a mechanism known as predictive processing. We may find ourselves worrying more, and jumping to conclusions when schemas are activated—the size of the Evaluation box has increased! This is accompanied by more activity in the "default mode network," which encompasses the areas of the brain that are active when we are daydreaming, planning for the future, thinking about the past, and having "I," "me," and "mine" thoughts. The default mode network is also more active when we are worrying and ruminating.

Finally, you'll notice that when the information processing system is in disequilibrium, the size of the fourth box, Co-emerging Body Sensations, is smaller than usual. This is because the valuable information contained in the co-emerging sensations is not being processed as effectively. Adaptive problem-solving decreases, leading to more reactivity, increasing the size of box 5. If this unbalanced state persists, it becomes our new way of being, as often occurs with chronic stress or anxiety.

Perhaps the following situation is familiar. Imagine that you are relaxing on your couch when you get a call from a friend you were supposed to call yesterday but didn't. If information is being processed in a state of *disequilibrium*, your attention is more likely to quickly shift from sensory perception (hearing the phone ring, feeling it vibrate) to thinking (I *should have called them yesterday. Now they're probably upset with me. I'm a bad friend. I'm a disappointment to everyone*). The "I," "me," and associated underlying belief patterns, or schemas, become prominent. These unhelpful thoughts and beliefs are accompanied by unpleasant co-emerging sensations, such as a tightness in the chest or a heavy sinking feeling in the lower abdomen.

What is our usual automatic next step? We don't answer the phone. We might even turn it off to ensure that we don't know if our friend is trying to call us back. And we might reach out for some means of distraction to soothe ourselves and forget about the situation. We do all of this to avoid feeling the unpleasant sensations that co-emerge with our thoughts, though we might be under the impression at the time that we are just avoiding speaking to our friend.

Figure 5 shows how this situation can be mapped onto the co-emergence model. We can see how decreased sensory perception is experienced—how quickly one's attention moves from the objective particulars of the situation, like the ringing phone, to subjective evaluations of it. We see how increased evaluation manifests as self-criticism, and as self-focused thoughts of "I" and "me," rather than thoughts of the friend and why they might be calling. Decreased awareness of co-emerging sensations is evident in the way one becomes less emotionally aware, and increased reactivity is evident in the habitual self-soothing behaviors.

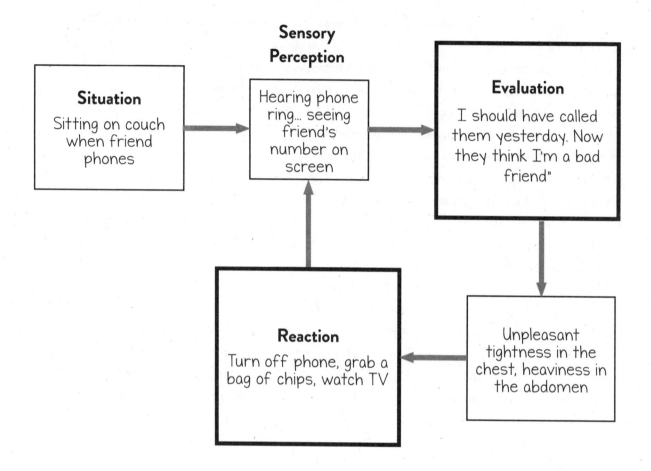

In week 3, you'll learn to map your own stressful and challenging experiences onto the co-emergence model of reinforcement using the Diary of Reactive Habits to explore and gain insight into your habitual thought and behavior patterns. For now, we'll take a look at how we can restore flexible equilibrium to a system of information processing that's become unbalanced.

## Developing Equanimity to Bring Back Equilibrium in Information Processing

Returning to a state of equilibrium—and along the way, alleviating symptoms of depression and anxiety—requires a novel approach to both pleasant and unpleasant co-emerging sensations. The key lies in replacing our habitual reactions to these sensations with the skill known as equanimity. While mindfulness centers on bringing an objective attention to our moment-to-moment internal experience, equanimity is a non-reactive and accepting attitude toward that experience, whether it is pleasant, unpleasant, or neutral. With equanimity, there is a genuine acceptance of our internal experience as it is arising in the present moment and a willingness to experience it just as it is.

Equanimity is instrumental in addressing depressive and anxiety symptoms. Picture this common scenario: a depressive or anxious thought arises, accompanied by co-emerging unpleasant sensations. This is expected, automatic, and very natural—and we can influence what happens next. Instead of avoiding these unpleasant sensations, we can turn towards them with equanimity. Equanimity entails a sincere willingness to feel sensations as they are, wholeheartedly, with unconditional acceptance, even if initially only for a few seconds! By intentionally choosing to welcome the feeling of unpleasantness in this way, we abstain from our typical reactive behaviors. Similarly, we can apply equanimity to pleasant sensations, preventing attachment or craving. This disrupts the cyclical patterns that often amplify and perpetuate depressive and anxiety symptoms.

Recent research underscores the effectiveness of equanimity and interoceptive awareness in combatting these symptoms (Wu et al. 2022). This becomes especially relevant for individuals grappling with concurrent anxiety and depression, as they are more avoidant of unpleasant sensations compared to individuals with depression alone (Ironside et al. 2023). Equanimity is a natural antidote to this kind of avoidance.

A common misunderstanding of equanimity is that it involves detachment from our feelings. In reality, numbing or disengaging from emotions is the opposite of equanimity—instead of feeling less, equanimity allows us to feel our emotions more deeply and with more acceptance. We will explore this in detail in weeks 3 and 4. Ultimately, mindfulness and equanimity will help you cope adaptively with distressing thoughts, be less emotionally reactive, make better choices, and increase social connections with supportive people.

Take a moment to complete the short equanimity questionnaire below, the Equanimity Scale-16. This will measure your equanimity level before you start MiCBT, which you can compare with later measurements to see how it increases over time.

## Equanimity Scale-16

Select the response that best describes how much you agree with each statement right at this moment, based on the scale below. Remember that there are no right or wrong answers.

*Strongly disagree = 1*    *Mildly disagree = 2*    *Agree and disagree equally = 3*

*Mildly agree = 4*    *Strongly agree = 5*

| | | | | | |
|---|---|---|---|---|---|
| 1. When I have distressing thoughts or images, I am able just to notice them without reacting. | 1 | 2 | 3 | 4 | 5 |
| 2. I approach each experience by trying to accept it, no matter whether it is pleasant or unpleasant. | 1 | 2 | 3 | 4 | 5 |
| 3. When I experience distressing thoughts and images, I am able to accept the experience. | 1 | 2 | 3 | 4 | 5 |
| 4. I can pay attention to what is happening in my body without disliking or wanting more of the feeling or sensation. | 1 | 2 | 3 | 4 | 5 |
| 5. When I notice my feelings, I have to act on them immediately. | 1 | 2 | 3 | 4 | 5 |
| 6. If I notice an unpleasant body sensation, I tend to worry about it. | 1 | 2 | 3 | 4 | 5 |
| 7. When I feel physical discomfort, I can't relax because I am never sure it will pass. | 1 | 2 | 3 | 4 | 5 |
| 8. I perceive my feelings and emotions without having to react to them. | 1 | 2 | 3 | 4 | 5 |
| 9. I remain present with sensations and feelings even when they are unpleasant. | 1 | 2 | 3 | 4 | 5 |
| 10. I notice that I need to react to whatever pops into my head. | 1 | 2 | 3 | 4 | 5 |
| 11. When I have distressing thoughts or images, I "step back" and am aware of the thought or image without getting taken over by it. | 1 | 2 | 3 | 4 | 5 |
| 12. I can't keep my mind calm and clear, especially when I feel upset or physically uncomfortable. | 1 | 2 | 3 | 4 | 5 |
| 13. I endeavor to cultivate calm and peace within me, even when everything appears to be constantly changing. | 1 | 2 | 3 | 4 | 5 |
| 14. I am impatient and can't stop my reactivity when faced with other people's emotions and actions. | 1 | 2 | 3 | 4 | 5 |
| 15. I am not able to tolerate discomfort. | 1 | 2 | 3 | 4 | 5 |
| 16. I am not able to prevent my reaction when someone is unpleasant. | 1 | 2 | 3 | 4 | 5 |

## Scoring

To calculate your total score:

### Step 1

For items 1, 2, 3, 4, 8, 9, 11, and 13, your item score is simply your response.

For items 5, 6, 7, 10, 12, 14, 15, and 16, reverse the score of your response as follows.

| Your Response | Reversed Score |
|:---:|:---:|
| 1 | 5 |
| 2 | 4 |
| 3 | 3 |
| 4 | 2 |
| 5 | 1 |

### Step 2

Add up all the scores and use the reversed scores for items 5, 6, 7, 10, 12, 14, 15, and 16.

This should give you a total score out of 80: _____ / 80

As a point of reference, the average score in the general population before equanimity training is 59/80.

You can find a downloadable version of the Equanimity Scale-16 at http://www.newharbinger.com/52571.

Adapted with permission from Rogers, H. T., A. G. Shires, and B. A. Cayoun. 2021. "Development and Validation of the Equanimity Scale-16." *Mindfulness* 12: 107–120. https://doi.org/10.1007/s12671-020-01503-6.

# Beginning Your Journey

In part 1 of this workbook, you've learned about the MiCBT approach to cultivating present-moment awareness, healthier thought patterns, and adaptive coping strategies. We reviewed how engaging in regular mindfulness practices and applying CBT techniques will help you progressively build resilience, foster emotional balance, and enhance your overall well-being. It's now time to embark on this transformative ten-week journey through the MiCBT program.

Part 2 of this workbook details the ten-week MiCBT program. Each week, you'll be guided through essential mindfulness exercises and CBT interventions designed to help you address anxiety and depression Remember, change takes time and commitment, so be patient with yourself as you navigate this path towards healing and self-discovery. Your dedication to this process will be rewarded with a renewed sense of clarity, inner tranquility, and emotional resilience. We look forward to supporting you on this journey.

## Audio Instructions

To ensure the precision and efficacy of your mindfulness meditation practice, we recommend using MiCBT-specific audio guides, voiced by Dr. Cayoun. Below, you'll find a comprehensive list of these resources, presented in MP3 format. You have the flexibility to either download these resources directly or stream them from the website at http://www.newharbinger.com/52571.

1. General Introduction (1:18)

2. Rationale for Training (10:56)

3. Introduction to Progressive Muscle Relaxation (PMR) (2:22)

4. Progressive Muscle Relaxation (14:00)

5. Introduction to Mindfulness of Breath (2:40)

6. Mindfulness of Breath (30:00)

7. Introduction to Body Scanning (1:41)

8. Body Scanning (31:31)

9. Practicing in Silence (3:24)

10. Introduction to the Mindfulness-based Interoceptive Exposure Task (MIET) (2:54)

11. The Mindfulness-based Interoceptive Exposure Task (6:05)

12. Introduction to Advanced Scanning Practices (2:44)

13. Symmetrical Scanning (30:00)

14. Introduction to Bipolar Exposure (1:05)

15. Bipolar Exposure Task (11:00)

16. Introduction to Partial Sweeping (1:35)

17. Partial Sweeping (30:00)

18. Introduction to Sweeping *en Masse* (1:46)

19. Sweeping *en Masse* (30:00)

20. Introduction to Transversal Scanning (1:20)

21. Transversal Scanning (30:00)

22. Introduction to Sweeping in Depth (01:00)

23. Sweeping in Depth (30:00)

24. Introduction to Loving-Kindness (3:12)

25. Loving-Kindness (8:11)

26. Maintenance Practice (44:56)

## Terms of Use of Audio Tracks

All audio files are copyrighted by Dr. Bruno A. Cayoun. This license grants the right to stream and download the audio files at http://www.newharbinger.com/52571 for private and domestic use. For example, you can, for your private use, copy recordings onto your tablet, smartphone or MP3 player, and copy legitimately acquired digital files onto a computer or CD to play in your stereo.

This license is limited to you, the purchaser of this book. This license does not grant the right to sell, give away, distribute, perform in public, or broadcast private copies, make private copies from an illegitimate recording (e.g., from a burnt CD or from peer-to-peer files), or share private copies online. Uploading or distributing music via the Internet without permission from the copyright owner will infringe copyright. (Similarly, this license grants the right to download and print the PDF forms located at http://www.newharbinger.com/52571 for your private and domestic use only.)

# Part 2

# The Program, Step by Step

# Cultivating Self-Care

This chapter introduces the practice of progressive muscle relaxation (PMR) to train the ability to relax while developing body awareness. PMR grounds you in the present moment, using the body as an anchor for attention. By being aware of our posture and movements during the day, we begin to move away from ruminating over the past and worrying about the future.

## Progressive Muscle Relaxation

MiCBT starts with PMR. Although it is not a mindfulness practice itself, it is a valuable tool for calming and relaxing the nervous system before starting mindfulness meditation. PMR was developed in the 1920s by an American physician (Jacobson 1942) and has been scientifically studied since the 1970s. There is evidence supporting its effectiveness in multiple conditions, including reducing symptoms of stress, anxiety, depression, and improving sleep.

### What Will I Be Learning?

We use PMR in MiCBT to help train several skills, including releasing tension from areas of the body as needed, and feeling more present, which supports mental calmness. In addition, PMR helps you learn an important skill: to be both relaxed *and* alert at the same time.

Sometimes we might feel a bit worried or anxious about paying attention to sensations in the body. This can occur, for example, if we've experienced persistent anxiety, trauma, or chronic pain. Relaxing can cause us to become more aware of worry, painful memories, or physical discomfort, and we instinctively would rather not feel these. However, avoidance is not an effective solution in the long term. In contrast, when practicing PMR, *we* are in control of contracting muscles and then letting the tension go, and so *we* feel in control of the sensations we're feeling, which brings a sense of reassurance and confidence.

## Committing to Self-Care

It can be a radical act to prioritize our well-being. For most of us, it will take careful thought and preparation to add these two fourteen-minute practices into our day. You may need to set your alarm twenty minutes earlier and rearrange your evening routines. If you live with others, you might need to tell them that you'll be unavailable at certain times. This is a great opportunity to become aware of unhelpful beliefs such as *I don't deserve to take time to do this for me*, or *Other people's needs are more important than mine*. A good way to motivate yourself is to look back at your success indicators in chapter 1. What are your hopes and goals for engaging in this program? Remind yourself why it's important to prioritize this practice and consider the change agreement you signed and the commitment to yourself you've made. Keep in mind that once you have practiced PMR twice daily for a few days, the results will be enough to keep you going—the benefits will speak for themselves.

### Recap: PMR Benefits

Training in PMR twice a day this week, you will learn to:

1. Allow your body to relax while remaining connected to your present moment experience.
2. Stay mentally alert while relaxed.
3. Prioritize time for self-care twice a day.
4. Identify and address any unhelpful thoughts about self-care (e.g., feeling guilty or worrying about wasting time).

## Applying Your Skills: Mindfulness of the Body

James Joyce once wrote that a character "lived at a little distance from his body" (1914). With anxiety and depression, it's easy to become lost in thoughts and disconnected from bodily experience. Sometimes this can be quite subtle, and other times it can be very obvious, and we may feel numb or dissociated. When this keeps up over time, as we described in chapter 2, areas of the brain involved in feeling sensations in the body become less active. Because joy, happiness, and other positive emotional experiences require feeling sensations in the body, this can leave us feeling "flat" and unmotivated. One of the simplest ways of beginning to reverse these changes in the brain is to repeatedly bring attention to our body position and movements during the day.

## What Is Mindfulness of the Body?

Mindfulness of the body is described in Buddhist psychology as the first of four "foundations" of mindfulness (Anālayo 2018). The other three are mindfulness of pleasant, unpleasant, and neutral body sensations, mindfulness of mental states (anger, peace, greed, etc.) and of mental phenomena, including thoughts. We introduced you to the second foundation of mindfulness in chapter 3, when we discussed the pleasant, unpleasant, and neutral tone of body sensations in box 4 of the CMR. We'll be exploring all four of these foundations of mindfulness over the next ten weeks together.

This week we begin working with mindfulness of the body by bringing attention to our posture and movement. We can be quite objective about the position of the body—are we sitting? Standing? Walking? Lying down? As you practice during the day, you might notice thoughts about body position, such as *Now I'm sitting*. Although it is normal to have thoughts about your experience, you don't need to think *I'm standing* to know that you are standing. You only need to feel it. By bringing mindfulness to feeling the body repeatedly throughout the day, over time, you can develop the ability to know the experience of sitting or standing directly, without the additional thoughts about it.

## Bringing Your Attention to the Present

Mindfulness of the body during the day assists us in remaining present with what is happening within and around us. When we feel depressed or anxious, it can feel especially difficult to be present with our partner, children, friends, and others to whom we want to pay full attention. Is this familiar to you? Our mind can get stuck in the past or in our anticipated future—anywhere but in the here and now! By using your body's movement and posture as an anchor for your attention, you train your mind to be present.

However, for this exercise to be consistent with training in mindfulness it is important that your awareness is untainted by judgments. You'll need to refrain from thoughts that "like" or "dislike" the body. It is neither too large nor too thin, neither too young nor too old, neither too attractive nor too unattractive. It is just a body. And it does not define who you are, as it—and you—will keep on changing over time!

# Remembering to Practice Mindfulness of the Body During the Day

One of the hardest things about practicing mindfulness as we go about our usual activities is remembering to do it! Here are a few ideas for how to remember to bring a non-judgemental attention to the body during the day, and space to write your own as well:

1.  Place sticky notes or other reminders in visible locations.

2.  Set reminders on your phone.

3.  Choose specific activities during which to bring attention to the position and movement of the body, like when walking in specific areas of your home or workplace, putting on clothes, or washing dishes.

Here is an example of a plan to help bring more mindfulness into the day:

| | |
|---|---|
| Sticky notes: | On the kitchen counter |
| | On the mirror in the bathroom |
| Reminder on my phone: | Every 30 minutes |
| Mindful of my body when: | I sit down and stand up |
| | I brush my teeth |

Write down your own mindfulness reminders below:

| | |
|---|---|
| Sticky notes: | |
| | |
| | |
| Reminder on my phone: | |
| Mindful of my body when: | |
| | |
| | |
| Other ideas: | |
| | |
| | |
| | |

And, once you've set up some mindfulness reminders—use them!

## This Week's Practice

During the PMR practice, you'll be guided to contract and relax groups of muscles throughout your body in a specific order. This practice is best done in a seated position, because one of the things we are training is being relaxed and alert at the same time, and our body associates lying down with sleeping. Audio track 4 provides detailed guidance for this practice.

By repeatedly bringing your awareness to the position and movements of your body, you'll also be building the helpful habit of keeping your mind in the present throughout the day!

## Daily Record of Progressive Muscle Relaxation Practice

| Day | Date | Morning Practice | Duration (Minutes) | Observations About My PMR Practice (E.g., felt contraction and then release of tension in some areas; drowsy/alert; peaceful/frustrated, etc.) | Evening Practice | Duration (Minutes) | Observations About My PMR Practice (E.g., felt contraction and then release of tension in some areas; drowsy/alert; peaceful/frustrated, etc.) |
|---|---|---|---|---|---|---|---|
| Day 1 | | yes / no | | | yes / no | | |
| Day 2 | | yes / no | | | yes / no | | |
| Day 3 | | yes / no | | | yes / no | | |
| Day 4 | | yes / no | | | yes / no | | |
| Day 5 | | yes / no | | | yes / no | | |
| Day 6 | | yes / no | | | yes / no | | |
| Day 7 | | yes / no | | | yes / no | | |

## Week 1 Checklist

At the end of the week, record your total number of PMR practices, out of a maximum of fourteen, as well as the number of days that you practiced mindfulness of body during the day.

- ☐ Progressive muscle relaxation: _____ / 14

   - ☐ Audio Tracks 1 to 3: for the first two practices only

   - ☐ Audio Track 4: listen with each PMR practice

   - ☐ Daily Record of Progressive Muscle Relaxation Practice

- ☐ Mindfulness of body throughout the day: _____ / 7

# When Should I Read the Next Chapter?

After you finish one week of PMR and mindfulness of the body, continue to the next chapter to begin mindfulness of breath practice. There is no need to read ahead. Completing one week of PMR and mindfulness of the body first will ensure your understanding of what you read at the beginning of week 2 is informed by your lived experience of these practices. Theory and practice are best learned at the same time, allowing one to inform the other.

# Improving and Controlling Your Attention

This week is the start of your formal mindfulness meditation practice, beginning with mindfulness of breath practice. Practicing with the audio guidance, you'll learn to cultivate a calm mind and see depressive and anxious thoughts for what they truly are—just thoughts! You will reduce worrying and rumination by applying these skills to unhelpful thoughts. And the skills you learn by concentrating on the breath this week will also be very helpful next week when you start practicing the next meditation method.

## Review of Last Week's Practices

How was your practice of progressive muscle relaxation last week? Were you able to practice twice a day? Could you feel the difference between tension and relaxation?

As you probably noticed, the mind can be distracted by many thoughts, even during relaxation practice! We are so used to being mentally stimulated every day, sometimes because our work requires significant mental effort, or because we are accustomed to worrying, or maybe we have developed a social media habit that we use to regulate how we feel. Because PMR does not directly address the busyness of the mind, we need to work with the thoughts themselves. We'll be using the mindfulness of breath practice this week to do just this.

Before we dive in, let's check in on how it went with establishing a routine of practicing twice daily.

### Addressing Challenges to Practicing Twice Daily

Mindfulness programs rely on regular practice, because this is how you strengthen beneficial connections in your brain to help manage distressing thoughts and emotions skillfully. If you practiced at least once a day last week, you can proceed with this week's practice.

However, we understand that establishing a consistent practice can be challenging, and it may be helpful to spend a few more days adjusting your routine to support you in practicing twice daily. The key is to recognize the following common challenges as they arise, and implement strategies to address them.

## Time

By far the most common challenge is thinking that we are too busy to practice. We can feel too busy with "more urgent things" than making time to look after ourselves, even when we know that improving our mental health will benefit not just ourselves but others around us. Whether it involves making time to cook healthy meals, exercise, or meditate, adding another healthy activity for self-care can sometimes feel like too much. One way to approach this is to identify an activity that is lower priority than your well-being and happiness and replace it with one that promotes self-care.

## Sleep

A frequent worry about practicing twice daily is whether we'll get enough sleep. This can especially apply to morning practice, when we might need to set our alarm thirty minutes earlier in order to add meditation to our routine. It might be helpful to know that people who practice mindfulness regularly report improved sleep quality, restfulness, and energy levels during the day (Black et al. 2015).

## Guilt

Guilt can also get in the way. Sometimes, it can feel self-indulgent to put aside thirty minutes twice daily "just for ourselves" when we know how much our partner has to do, or how much our children want our attention. We may feel selfish practicing meditation if we've also made time for yoga, physical exercise, or creative activities; thoughts can arise that we should be working or with our family instead. To help overcome this, consider that your mental well-being also needs attention, and remind yourself why you decided to do this program.

To identify these potential challenges as they might manifest in your own life, please fill in the table below. If you answer "yes" for any of the limiting thoughts or beliefs, write down what the *actual* potential costs and benefits would be of meditating twice daily. Add one or more of your own limiting thoughts or beliefs in the last row if helpful.

| Limiting Thoughts or Beliefs | Yes/No | Potential Costs of Practicing 30 Minutes Twice Daily | Potential Benefits of Practicing 30 Minutes Twice Daily |
|---|---|---|---|
| I won't have time to do it. | | | |
| I worry about not sleeping enough. | | | |
| I feel guilty about caring for myself. | | | |
| Other examples | | | |

Once you're done with the exercise, consider: has looking at the potential benefits and costs of regular meditation practice changed your willingness to practice, or did it help you refine your strategies for implementing a twice-daily practice?

# Mindfulness of Breath

It is time now to practice the third and fourth foundation of mindfulness—that is, mindfulness of thoughts and mental states, using mindfulness of breath. You will learn to keep attention on your breath from moment to moment. This can require significant effort at first, and the calming, restful effects—it's called "calm-abiding meditation" for good reason—become increasingly apparent once skills are established. Although you may initially be *more* aware of thoughts while practicing, as your attention regulation skills improve, you will progressively feel freer from distressing thoughts. This is usually achievable within the first week, given consistent twice-daily practice that follows the method we'll outline. Let's look in more detail at the important skills you'll be developing.

## Attention Regulation

Mindfulness of breath meditation is a concentration training which develops three essential aspects of our attention: sustaining attention, response inhibition, and shifting attention.

### Sustaining Attention

The core of this practice involves keeping your attention on your breath, despite the draw of other sensations in the body, sounds, or thoughts. Recognizing the moment our attention has been pulled away from the chosen object of attention is a pivotal skill in itself. This applies to our daily life, where being able to promptly notice that we are experiencing anxious or depressive thoughts empowers us to not become caught up in them.

### Response Inhibition

This skill involves preventing our automatic reactivity to thoughts and sensations. Instead of passively following every thought that arises during meditation, we notice thoughts as just thoughts and learn to gently decline their invitations. It may seem surprising that we need to "take charge" of what we think, but it is not a form of harsh control. Rather, not engaging in habitual thoughts that contribute to depression or anxiety is like choosing to not eat a food item that we know isn't beneficial for us.

It can feel like a huge effort at first, as we're generally used to thinking whatever comes into our minds—we can even feel compelled to finish a thought that we've started, simply out of habit! In mindfulness of breath meditation, we develop response inhibition by systematically "declining" to engage with a thought each time one appears. Through this we prevent the thinking of it. In other words, we inhibit our previously learned response of thinking whatever comes into our mind.

## *Shifting Attention*

The third essential skill is the ability to deliberately shift our attention to focus on a different thing or task. Have you noticed how difficult it can be to refocus attention when you are caught up in worrying? Brain areas used for rumination connect themselves more strongly every time worrying occurs, making this habit increasingly difficult to shake. During mindfulness of breath, every time attention moves to a thought becomes a wonderful opportunity to practice this skill of shifting attention—in this case, back to the breath.

# Increasing the Effectiveness of Your Practice

In this section, we'll cover four important elements that can increase the effectiveness of your practice: posture, your surroundings, timing, and refraining from intoxicants. Although these are not prescriptive, we very much encourage you to consider applying them to optimize the benefits of your practice.

## Posture

During meditation, your posture matters. Sitting with your eyes closed and your neck and back straight will help your attention remain sharp and clearly focused. Slouching, on the other hand, will encourage drowsiness and could contribute to back pain. Some people prefer to sit on a chair; others prefer sitting cross-legged on the floor. Either is fine, provided your neck and back remain straight.

To assist with maintaining a straight posture, it is best to have your knees lower than your hips. This protects the natural lower curve of the spine. If you're sitting on a chair, this may require elevating the height of the seat by placing a cushion or folded towel on it. Try not to lean against the back of the chair, as the slumped posture that results is likely to contribute to drowsiness and lack of focus. If you choose to sit on the floor, use a higher cushion, bolster, or firm pillows It is best to avoid sofas and armchairs as they are usually quite low, which makes keeping your lower back straight more difficult.

## Room and Surroundings

At this early stage of learning meditation practice, it is most productive to practice indoors. Sitting on the beach warmed by the sun while feeling a soft wind caressing your face may be great, but it also comes with many distractions. The less your senses are stimulated by the environment the better, at least at this early stage of practice. This is because we're learning to become aware of internal experiences, and being distracted by external stimulation through our five senses delays progress.

The room in which you meditate is most conducive to efficient practice if the lighting is not too bright or too dark, the temperature is not too hot, and it is relatively quiet. Even with reasonable precautions to limit distracting sounds, some sounds will always occur, many of them outside of your control. You can use these sounds as part of your practice by relating to them as moment-to-moment reminders to notice where your attention is placed.

## Time of Day

To optimize progress, practice twice daily, once in the morning and again in the late afternoon or early evening, spacing out the sessions. Because shorter and frequent practices enhance skill development, two thirty-minute sessions are preferable to a single hour-long session. If you are constrained by your schedule, closer intervals are acceptable. Aim for your second session before dinner, and avoid practicing on a full stomach to prevent drowsiness. Practice earlier in the evening if possible, as tiredness can impede late-night sessions. In the end, regular practice is crucial. If "optimal" conditions are not available, that's okay, do it whenever you can!

# A Clear Mind for Good Practice

Training to become more mindful of our experience requires the ability to pay careful attention. If you practice while under the influence of alcohol or other substances, it will be difficult to focus clearly, and your practice will not be as productive because most substances interfere with response inhibition. If you continue to use alcohol or drugs during this program, please reduce the amount, and consume them only *after* your meditation practice. As you progress with your practice, you may find you need less of the substance to feel relieved or satisfied.

Once you've organized a place and time to practice, you're ready to start!

# Mindfulness of Breath Practice

Guided by the thirty-minute audio instructions, start by sitting with an upright posture and focusing attention on the breath coming in and going out of the nostrils. You might feel the movement and temperature of the air inside and below the nostrils, above the upper lip.

It is important that you breathe in your usual, natural way, rather than controlling the breath. The breath may be deep or shallow, fast or slow; just notice and accept it as it is. Although sometimes controlling the breath can be an effective way to relax the mind and body when anxious, doing so during this practice would interfere with training the three components of attention mentioned above and delay benefits. This is because controlling the breath requires thinking about it, which in turn interferes with the natural flow of spontaneous thoughts. Thoughts, rather than the breath, are the real point of interest for us when it comes to reducing anxiety.

Although the intention is to keep your attention focused on the breath, attention will naturally repeatedly be drawn to thoughts, especially when first starting to practice. Don't get frustrated. This is normal; it's just the way the mind works. When attention moves to a thought, gently remember that it is only "thinking"—even though some of the thoughts may try to convince you that they are very urgent or important and need to be attended to at that moment! Patiently, with a kind attitude, shift your attention back to the breath without delay to prevent becoming caught up in the thoughts. Remember that we're only using the breath as an anchor point in order to more clearly observe this bounty of thoughts and learn about the habitual activity of the mind.

We usually practice with eyes closed to minimize visual distractions. However, sometimes this can be anxiety provoking, such as when there has been a history of trauma. Whatever the reason, if this happens, it can be helpful to close your eyes halfway and direct your gaze downward, about six feet in front of your knees. This will let you see where you are and know that you are safe, while still minimizing distractions. As your confidence improves, you can close your eyes a little more in each practice session.

Mindfulness of breath practice this week is not only beneficial in its own right, but it also trains prerequisite skills for beginning body scanning next week.

## Five Common Challenges During Mindfulness Practice

As your practice for this week continues, you'll likely encounter a few challenges, such as aversion to what feels unpleasant, attachment to what feels pleasant, and perhaps a sense of drowsiness or dullness that makes it hard to stay consistently engaged. Understanding these common experiences can help us learn about habits of the mind, which are present whether we are meditating or going about our day. By recognizing these challenges and learning to relate to them differently, we can use them as opportunities to train mindfulness skills rather than seeing them as obstacles.

### Aversion

During practice, we might find ourselves reacting negatively to an unpleasant aspect of the experience. We may become impatient with our busy mind that seems to refuse to stay focused. We can have a painful memory and start to feel resentful toward someone. We can also find ourselves being irritated by an itch on the nose! Driven by aversion, we react, scratching the itch to stop the unpleasant sensations.

Although reacting to discomfort through aversion may provide temporary relief, it increases frustration in the long run, as our struggle with the unpleasantness compounds the initial discomfort.

We can best approach both the initial unpleasant sensations as well as any aversion toward them by focusing attention on the unpleasant sensations in the center of the area of greatest intensity, with curiosity and equanimity while refraining from reactivity. Becoming tolerant and accepting of momentary unpleasant sensations will allow them to pass more rapidly.

## Attachment

During practice, you might also encounter various pleasant body sensations and mental states, such as warmth, tingling, ease, peace, or calmness. It is natural to want these experiences to continue, but attachment to them can lead to disappointment, disheartenment, or doubt about your ability to progress when they inevitably change.

The issue isn't the enjoyment of pleasantness itself, but rather the craving for it to continue. This craving results in frustration or disappointment when the pleasant experience ceases or changes. It is essential to recognize that all experiences are temporary in nature and to learn to appreciate and enjoy them without clinging to them.

During meditation, it is also common to find ourselves getting caught up in pleasurable thoughts about future events or pleasant memories, and the accompanying subtle pleasant sensations in the body. Our natural reaction is to want more of these sensations, leading us to continue to think about past experiences or get caught up in planning our next enjoyable activity.

To address attachment and craving, start by recognizing when you're becoming attached to a pleasant experience or desiring something to be different or somehow "better" than it is right now. Be curious about how this attachment manifests and its connection to sensations in the body. Appreciate and enjoy the pleasant sensations while they are present, but don't mourn their passing or strive to prolong them. Then, just like with other sensations, move your attention away from them, and any accompanying thoughts or images, by refocusing on the intended object of attention.

## Dullness and Drowsiness

Developing mindfulness skills effectively requires making the most of your meditation time. Drowsiness can hinder progress, so addressing its potential causes, such as sleep deprivation, is crucial. Dull attention can manifest in many ways, such as:

1. A dozy warmth

2. Increased time taken to recognize when attention has moved off the intended focus

3. Feeling unmotivated or lazy

4. Starting to dream

5. Nodding off

To minimize drowsiness before practicing, take these precautions:

1. Practice before eating, particularly if eating a large or heavy meal.

2. Ensure the room temperature and light levels promote alertness; avoid overly dark or warm settings.

3. Maintain a straight back and neck while sitting, without leaning against the back of your chair or against something else if you are sitting on the floor.

4. Refrain from intoxicants before meditating.

If drowsiness persists despite these precautions, try these steps in this order:

1. Breathe deeper and slightly faster for up to a minute to sharpen sensations and wake the mind, but without hyperventilating.

2. Open your eyes slightly, focusing on the floor six feet in front of your knees, allowing light into your eyes, yet without visual distractions. After a minute or two, resume practicing with eyes closed.

3. Practice in a standing position, supported by a wall, for a few minutes before resuming sitting.

4. Rinse your face with cold water and restart in the sitting posture.

5. Go on a brisk walk for two to three minutes, then return to sitting.

6. If drowsiness remains, try sitting cross-legged for a short while, if you're not doing so already, to promote wakefulness—the mild discomfort you may feel will help you stay alert.

7. Engage in moderate to vigorous exercise for ten to fifteen minutes before starting your practice.

By implementing these strategies, you can counteract drowsiness and cultivate a more focused and effective mindfulness practice.

## Agitation and Restlessness

You might encounter agitation or restlessness, which often manifest as physical discomfort, an urge to shift or move, mental anxiety, or even frustration with ourselves, others, or the practice. Our mind may create narratives in an effort to explain this restlessness, making us believe that altering our surroundings or mental state will bring relief. However, reacting to restlessness with more restlessness only creates more agitation. To approach restlessness or agitation mindfully:

1.  *Acknowledge the experience:* Recognize the presence of restlessness or agitation. Observe them without avoidance or judgment. See them for what they are.

2.  *Focus on the breath:* Your breath can serve as an anchor. Notice any changes in your breath associated with agitation and continue focusing on it for a few minutes. As your breath settles, your mind will follow.

3.  *Observe the mind-body connection:* Use this experience to understand how restlessness in the mind affects your body. By becoming aware of this interplay, you can develop a deeper understanding of the relationship between mind and body.

## Doubt and Confusion

While some doubt during mindfulness meditation can lead to helpful inquiry and result in deeper understanding, persistent doubt can hinder progress, so addressing it quickly is crucial. There are three main types of doubt:

1.  *Doubt about the technique:* Trust is key to resolving this type of doubt. Learn about the research demonstrating that mindfulness is an effective treatment for depression and anxiety. Remember that meditation practice has a long history of success.

2.  *Doubt about your teachers:* Establishing trust in the teachers can enhance your commitment and adherence to instructions, helping you obtain the expected benefits. Consider the teachers' experience, dedication, and connection to a knowledgeable and respected lineage of teachers.

3.  *Doubt about oneself:* Self-doubt can jeopardize your progress in both meditation and other areas of life. It is essential to develop a trust in your ability to overcome obstacles, and to grow and succeed. To work with self-doubt during practice, notice that self-doubting thoughts are based on "I" and "me," rather than the practice. Observe doubting thoughts as mere thoughts,

without taking them personally. As you consistently reappraise self-doubting thoughts without identifying with them, they will decrease in frequency and intensity, and their grip on you will lessen.

# Seeing Thoughts as Just Mental Events

Developing mindfulness skills involves recognizing that thoughts are just mental events, not reality itself. Subconsciously, we may believe that we *are* our thoughts. The more we identify with thoughts, especially when feeling emotional, the more difficult it is to relinquish them and refocus on the breath. As we learn to let them pass, it becomes clearer that thoughts are *just* thoughts, mental events that arise and pass away.

Thoughts arise spontaneously for several reasons. One obvious one is because of our senses: hearing a truck may make you think of a truck, or feeling cold may remind you of a previous time that you felt this cold. Our thoughts, cued by thoughts about the past, can quickly switch to ones about the future, because our brains are constantly making predictions about what we will experience in the future based on our prior knowledge and experiences. Thoughts about possible outcomes of future conversations or planning future events are examples of this kind of predictive processing.

Thoughts also emerge for three other important reasons: the recency effect, frequency effect, and co-emergence effect. Understanding these causes of spontaneous thoughts will support you in recognizing them as impermanent and impersonal mental events. These three processes are continually at play whether we are meditating or not, but in the context of our daily activities we usually don't notice them as much—except perhaps when trying to fall asleep!

## Recency Effect

The *recency* effect is the increased likelihood that thoughts related to recent experiences or topics you've been thinking about recently will arise. For instance, if you enjoyed a pleasant walk home from work today, you're more likely to have thoughts about this walk during your evening meditation than about a similar walk a month ago.

## Frequency Effect

The *frequency* effect is that regularly occurring thoughts or topics are more likely to resurface. When we repeatedly think about a topic, our brain's memory networks related to this topic strengthen, facilitating these thoughts' reoccurrence. For example, if you have been having frequent ruminative thoughts about a specific family member, it's likely that thoughts about this family member will occur during meditation without prompting.

## Co-Emergence Effect

Over the course of our lives, pleasant and unpleasant sensations that we experience in the body are stored deep in memory, along with memories of the situation. Later, when we feel similar sensations, even if we are not consciously aware of them, memories of these past events are triggered. You may observe this *co-emergence effect* during your meditation practice—thoughts related to events that occurred years ago, even events from early childhood, may arise, all because a sensation of similar temperature, mass, motion, or density was felt! Mindfulness meditators often report having all sorts of childhood memories arise, including some that may seem random or strange, like those we would have in dreams. Once we are more acquainted with the practice, we can make sense of the apparent randomness.

# Applying Your Skills: Mindfulness of Thoughts in Daily Life

Meditating according to specific and precise instructions leads to beneficial changes in the brain that support us in making changes in our lives. In MiCBT, we accelerate this process by immediately applying the skills learned during meditation directly to our everyday activities. This produces rapid benefits, often in a single week. This week, we apply mindfulness of thoughts and mental states throughout the day to help us cultivate beneficial thoughts and discourage unhelpful ones.

An unhelpful thought, desire, or action is one that promotes unhappiness or dissatisfaction, whereas a helpful thought has a reduced probability of causing suffering.

Differentiating helpful thoughts from unhelpful thoughts is an important skill. It allows us to make better choices in the way we think, and therefore feel, in daily life. Unhelpful thoughts tend to co-emerge with more intense body sensations and are therefore more likely to lead to reactive behaviors. Helpful, wholesome thoughts tend to be less associated with intense body sensations. This also means that they are less likely to result in reactivity. As your mindfulness practice develops and you feel sensations even more clearly, it will become increasingly apparent whether a specific thought is helpful or not.

If you recall the discussion about suffering in chapter 2, reacting with craving for pleasant sensations and aversion to unpleasant ones is a significant source of suffering. As this happens much more frequently with unhelpful thoughts, we are much better off thinking in helpful ways, irrespective of the circumstances we are in. Developing the ability to choose skillful, helpful thoughts also increases our confidence and sense of agency over our lives.

## Practice Instructions

Throughout the day, you will be practicing mindfulness of thoughts and mental states. To this end, do your best to check in frequently on the type of thoughts that you are having.

Are they helpful or unhelpful?

### Disengaging from Unhelpful Thoughts

When you notice that you aren't having any unhelpful thoughts, continue to keep them at bay! Avoid inviting them in. For example, when we're accustomed to worrying, it can sometimes feel reassuring to start worrying again—we might be worried that we're forgetting something important to worry about! Do your best to not engage with any unhelpful thoughts.

When you notice that an unhelpful thought *is* present, use the three key skills you are practicing during meditation: notice that this is *just* a thought, inhibit the usual response of continuing to think it, and bring your attention back to the task at hand. This is a very helpful skill in reducing rumination, obsessions, self-critical thoughts, and other unhelpful thoughts during the day—and it can require vigilance.

Just as when we're weeding unwanted plants out of a large garden, this process takes time. And often, even as we're weeding, new weeds will begin to grow. It's the same with unhelpful thoughts. There is no doubt that your continued effort will bear fruit, but like a patient gardener who remains confident even when weeds are strong and tenacious, you need to be patient and self-assured when the task is difficult. Do your best to prevent thoughts of discouragement (which, it may help to keep in mind, are also *just thoughts*!).

### Cultivating Beneficial Thoughts

A similar approach applies to helpful thoughts. Whenever you examine your mind and notice that a helpful thought is *not* present, you can do your best to create one. This could be a thought steeped in gratitude, love, or compassion for someone else or for yourself. It can be related to feeling happy for someone else's success, achievement, or happiness. It can also be about feeling content in the present moment. The nature of the mind is to think; we might as well choose what it is that we're thinking! Just as we can plant the seeds we wish to grow after we weed unwanted plants out of our garden, we can actively nurture and intentionally think the thoughts we wish to cultivate after withdrawing attention from the ones that are unhelpful.

When practicing mindfulness of thoughts during the day, if you find that a helpful thought is present, you might work to keep it there, nourish it, make it last or grow. For example, if you realize that you're feeling good about how your day is going, you may think a little further about the consistent effort you are making to achieve this (an example of gratitude). Remember, wholesome thoughts create a wholesome mind, and a wholesome mind creates contentment!

Below you'll find a log for tracking your practice of mindfulness of thoughts during the day, if you find it useful. You can also download a printable version of this resource at http://www.newharbinger.com/52571.

## Tracking My Mindfulness of Thoughts in Daily Life Practice

| Date | Example of Unhelpful Thought | Example of Beneficial Thought |
|------|------------------------------|-------------------------------|
|      |                              |                               |
|      |                              |                               |
|      |                              |                               |
|      |                              |                               |
|      |                              |                               |
|      |                              |                               |
|      |                              |                               |

## This Week's Practice

This week you'll be practicing the thirty-minute mindfulness of breath meditation twice daily using the audio guidance on track 6. It is beneficial to listen to the brief introduction on track 5 at least twice. As in week 1, document your practice in the "Daily Record" worksheet in this chapter. There is no need to continue practicing PMR going forward, though you can return to it in the future as an additional practice if you choose.

Remind yourself to practice mindfulness of thoughts throughout the day, refraining from thinking those that are harmful, and allowing those that are beneficial to you.

---

## Week 2 Checklist

☐ Mindfulness of breath:  _____ / 14 practice sessions

  ☐ Audio Track 5: listen for the first two practices only

  ☐ Audio Track 6: listen with each practice

  ☐ Daily Record of Mindfulness of Breath Practice

☐ Mindfulness of thoughts during the day

---

## When Should I Read the Next Chapter?

As explained in the previous chapter, it is better to not read ahead; once you've practiced mindfulness of breath for one full week, continue to the next chapter to begin mindfulness of body sensations using "body scanning."

## Daily Record of Mindfulness of Breath Practice

| Day | Date | Morning Practice | Duration (Minutes) | Response Inhibition Rate from 1 to 10 how frequently you were able to notice distractions and bring attention back to the breath. 1 = once or twice; 10 = almost all the time | Evening Practice | Duration (Minutes) | Response Inhibition Rate from 1 to 10 how frequently you were able to notice distractions and bring attention back to the breath. 1 = once or twice; 10 = almost all the time |
|---|---|---|---|---|---|---|---|
| Day 1 | | yes / no | | | yes / no | | |
| Day 2 | | yes / no | | | yes / no | | |
| Day 3 | | yes / no | | | yes / no | | |
| Day 4 | | yes / no | | | yes / no | | |
| Day 5 | | yes / no | | | yes / no | | |
| Day 6 | | yes / no | | | yes / no | | |
| Day 7 | | yes / no | | | yes / no | | |

# Recognizing Emotions and Preventing Reactivity

This week, we explore the key role of body sensations in managing emotions, especially when dealing with depression and anxiety. You'll learn what the basic building blocks of emotions are and use this deeper understanding of emotional reactivity to address intense emotions constructively. Practicing "unilateral body scanning" to develop equanimity will lay the foundation for emotion regulation through training non-reactivity and acceptance of body sensations and improve your resilience during difficult situations.

## Review of Last Week's Practices

Reflecting on the past week, how did your mindfulness of breath practice progress? Were you able to notice thoughts quickly when they entered the mind? Were you able to refocus attention on the breath soon after? This is not an easy skill to develop, but it improves over time.

A common reason for finding it difficult to focus on the breath is insufficient practice. Sometimes we simply need more practice to develop the skills, especially if we were not able to practice at least twelve times this last week. If you are finding it challenging to maintain focus on your breath for even two to three breaths in a row, consider spending another week on mindfulness of breath, practicing in silence for the whole thirty minutes this time; practicing without audio guidance will help increase alertness. This time spent learning to notice when attention has moved away from the breath and then deliberately refocusing on the breath will yield many benefits in the coming weeks.

If you have been able to regularly focus on the breath for seven to ten consecutive breaths, i.e., about thirty seconds, during your recent thirty-minute meditations, you are ready to begin the practice of body scanning this week, and cultivate mindfulness of body sensations.

# Mindfulness of Body Sensations

This week you'll be practicing unilateral body scanning using detailed audio instructions. Body scanning develops our ability to feel both intense and subtle sensations in the body with greater objectivity and less reactivity. Through this process, we become aware of the intimate relationship between body sensations, thoughts and the ways in which they combine to create emotions.

## How Do We Experience Emotions?

When we're feeling an emotion, how do we know we're feeling it? This is an important question not to be taken for granted. Let's examine how we experience an emotion in a step-by-step logical manner.

1.  Given that an emotion is something we feel, we must feel it somewhere.

2.  The only place we can feel anything is in our body.

3.  Therefore, emotions can only be felt in the body in the form of sensations.

Let's test this. For example, how do you know that you feel anger when you're feeling angry? Where in your body does it manifest?

_____

How do you know that you feel fear when you're feeling afraid or anxious?

_____

How do you know that you feel sadness when you're feeling sad?

_____

Many people experience sadness as a heaviness somewhere in the body and perhaps a lack of energy. And they experience fear or anxiety in the form of a faster heartbeat, constriction in the chest or abdomen, and so on. This applies to all emotions and is the reason that we call body sensations the "building blocks of emotion" in emotion science (Barrett 2006).

# The Role of Body Scanning in Emotion Regulation

Since all emotions are experienced through body sensations, being able to feel and accept sensations makes it much easier to accept emotions. Beginning this week, you'll be focusing your twice daily practice on scanning the body, using progressively more demanding scanning techniques each week, to recognize emotions as they manifest in the body and to accept these sensations as they are.

Whether sensations in the body are caused by ambient temperature, posture, emotion, or other cause, the intention is to feel them, cultivate equanimity by accepting them without reactivity, and then move attention to the next part of the body to do the same. Through practicing this twice a day, and every day for several weeks, *all* body sensations progressively become acceptable.

We can bring the same skills to feeling and accepting sensations associated with emotional intensity during daily life. This is how we learn to regulate emotions with mindfulness meditation. Using the audio instructions for unilateral body scanning, you'll develop this skill a little more each day, noticing that while emotional reactivity may still arise, its duration decreases. When your skills are well developed, difficult emotions will be less intense and last a very short period of time.

# Feeling Without Reacting: The Key Role of Equanimity

Equanimity is central to the practice of body scanning. As discussed in chapter 3, equanimity is the ability to remain unperturbed by what we experience in our body and mind, combined with a willingness to experience it, whether it is pleasant, unpleasant, or neutral.

Equanimity has been researched by colleagues in different parts of the world (e.g., Hadash et al. 2016; Juneau 2020). In our own research (Rogers, Shires, and Cayoun 2021), we found that equanimity is composed of two elements: "non-reactivity" and "experiential acceptance."

## Non-Reactivity

*Non-reactivity* refers to preventing habitual reactivity to experiences, whether they are pleasant or unpleasant. As summarized in the co-emergence model of reinforcement, we often react with attachment when the experience is pleasant and with aversion when the experience is unpleasant. Reacting is best understood as "re-enacting" an unhelpful way of responding that we have learned in the past. In the past, we may have behaved in certain ways to get more of what we wanted and avoid what we didn't want. Over time, these behaviors turn into automatic responses and subconscious habits. In many ways, reacting automatically means we are living in the past, at the cost of missing the valuable reality of the present moment. Non-reactivity gives us the mental space to examine our *actual* internal experience as it's happening.

## Experiential Acceptance

"Acceptance," in this context, refers to the ability to accept an *internal* experience, such as a thought or sensation in the body. This is known as *experiential acceptance*. With the addition of equanimity, it goes beyond mere tolerance, and is not limited to an intellectual understanding. Instead, it involves a turning towards, a welcoming of the thought as a thought or the sensation as a sensation, as it is in the moment. There is no wish or hidden agenda that doing so will cause the sensation to lessen, go away if it is unpleasant, or prolong it if it is pleasant.

Importantly, experiencing a thought with equanimity does not in any way condone its content, or indicate agreement or disagreement—after all, it is just a thought! Acceptance also does not refer to passively accepting *external* circumstances such as domestic violence, gender inequality, social injustice, and other situations that create suffering and need to be proactively addressed.

### Equanimity with Painful Memories

What if, during meditation practice, we experience a painful memory and even feel unpleasant sensations co-emerging in the body with the memory? What do we do then? We turn towards the associated sensations with non-reactivity and a welcoming acceptance. By bringing equanimity even to potentially difficult internal experiences, we can observe them for what they are, just memories, thoughts, and body sensations that arise to pass away.

Accepting the embodied experience and emotional pain of this memory with equanimity also means that we are not avoiding or denying it. It is the first step to developing an accurate understanding of what that discomfort is made of, how the unpleasant sensations actually feel in the body, and how long the discomfort really lasts when we don't add reactivity to it. People are often very surprised that fully accepting unpleasant sensations, rather than avoiding or catastrophizing them, allows them to subside rapidly. We will discuss this in more detail in the next chapter, as week 4 focuses on developing equanimity.

## Unilateral Body Scanning

With this week's practice of *unilateral body scanning*, you'll be learning to feel sensations in the body in a systematic way, with equanimity, as well as observe the relationship between thoughts and sensations. Research has shown that people with anxiety and depression who ruminate a lot and are not able to feel body sensations well tend to experience more distress (Khalsa et al. 2018). By practicing body scanning, you'll be taking a big step towards reducing your distress.

## Practice Instructions

When you begin unilateral body scanning, you'll start by focusing at the top of your head on a spot about two to three inches in diameter for about ten seconds. As soon as you feel a sensation in the area you are scanning, move your attention to another small area next to the one you were just focusing on. The movement of attention is vertical, moving from the top of your head to the tips of your toes, and back to the top of your head. The audio instructions will guide you through the rest of the body, part by part.

During body scanning practice, we have a unique opportunity to offer a very different kind of response to unpleasant sensations. Instead of automatically doing something to lessen or change them—such as shifting posture, opening our eyes to look at the time, allowing ourselves to daydream, and so on—we practice equanimity. By maintaining an equanimous attitude toward sensations, whether pleasant or unpleasant, reactivity to sensations gradually diminishes (in a process called *generalized interoceptive desensitization*). With ongoing accurate practice, you'll notice that your equanimous attitude during meditation will progressively transfer to your daily experiences. This is a major achievement, because symptoms of depression and anxiety cannot coexist with equanimity.

As a beginner, it's normal to only feel sensations in certain areas, with much of the body feeling "blank." Be patient and persistent. This is the reality in this moment, in this part of the body. When you encounter a blank spot, pause and focus on that area for about thirty seconds, remaining attentive and equanimous. Accept the current absence of sensation, knowing that this too will change! If no sensation appears, maintain equanimity for the full thirty seconds and then move on to the next area confidently. If a sensation arises, proceed to the next spot without delay, before the thirty seconds have passed. Being aware informs you, and being equanimous transforms you!

# Applying Your Skills: Diary of Reactive Habits

The Diary of Reactive Habits is based on the co-emergence model of reinforcement, explained in chapter 3, and is used to apply our understanding of the relationship between thoughts, sensations, and reactivity to situations we encounter in daily life.

Remember that difficult situations can take two forms: circumstances external to us (e.g., being misunderstood by a family member, arriving late to a meeting, witnessing an accident, feeling tense around a friend or colleague, hearing a neighbor playing loud music late at night) or our own internal thoughts, feelings, and sensations (e.g., having a nightmare, experiencing pain in our body, remembering a stressful situation, worrying about something that will happen next week, or being afraid of becoming anxious or depressed). The examples below are of a difficult external and internal situation, respectively.

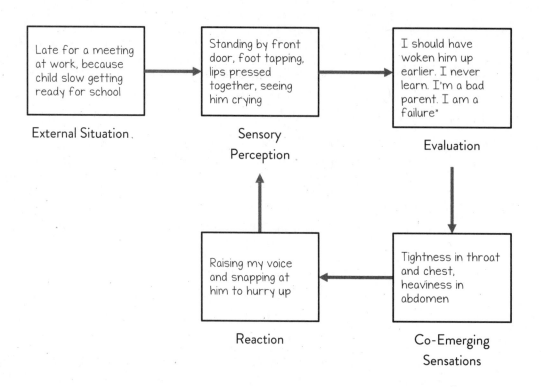

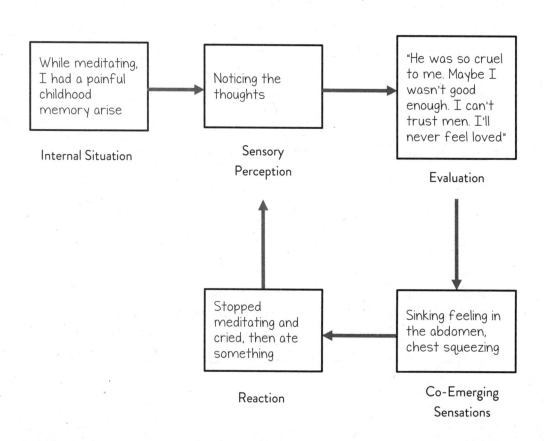

Now it's your turn. Use the Diary of Reactive Habits worksheet (also available at http://www.newhar binger.com/52571) to work through a difficult external or internal situation you experienced recently. Fill in the five components of your experience at the time.

Afterward, take some notes about your experience. Were you able to distinguish between the five components of experience, or was it challenging?

_____

_____

_____

_____

_____

_____

_____

_____

_____

_____

_____

_____

_____

_____

*Diary of Reactive Habits*

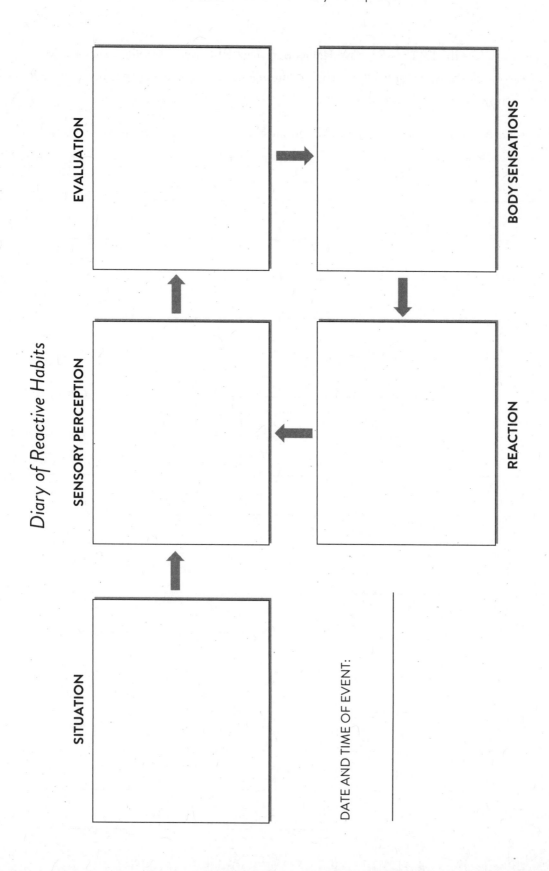

**EVALUATION**

**BODY SENSATIONS**

**SENSORY PERCEPTION**

**REACTION**

**SITUATION**

DATE AND TIME OF EVENT: _____

If it was difficult, just keep trying. The more you practice body scanning, the easier it will become to discern which aspects of your experience are represented in which box of the Diary of Reactive Habits.

## This Week's Practice

During unilateral body scanning twice daily this week, remember the emphasis on equanimity—we are practicing accepting sensations as they present themselves, from moment to moment. As with previous weeks, complete the Daily Record worksheet to track your practice, keep yourself accountable, and chart changes in your practice as they occur.

Also, after your first and last body scanning practices this week, use the Interoceptive Awareness Indicator, coloring in the parts of the silhouette where you felt any type of body sensation during your most recent practice. This gives you a visual representation of how much of the body you are feeling sensations in. You can also calculate the actual percentage of your interoceptive awareness as per the following instructions: The silhouette contains 100 boxes for the front of the body and 100 for the back. For each side, count each box that you have colored in as 1 percent interoceptive awareness. Once you have a total number of boxes counted for the front of the body, do the same for the back. Add the total number of boxes counted for the front and back, and divide that number by 2 to obtain your average percentage of interoceptive awareness and record it under the silhouette. You'll likely notice a significant increase in body awareness from the beginning to the end of the week!

Another copy of the Diary of Reactive Habits follows, and you can download additional copies from the website for this book. We encourage you to complete this exercise several times this week, as soon as you can after a stressful situation has occurred. This will allow you to become very familiar with the relationships between evaluative thoughts, co-emerging sensations, and reactions, and to be able to see these relationships unfold in "real time." We'll continue to build on this exercise next week when we introduce the mindfulness-based interoceptive exposure task (MIET).

# Week 3 Checklist

☐  Unilateral body scanning: _____ /14

    ☐  Audio Track 7: listen for the first two practices only

    ☐  Audio Track 8: listen with each practice

    ☐  Daily Record of Unilateral Body Scanning Practice

☐  Interoceptive Awareness Indicator

    ☐  After first body scanning this week

    ☐  After last body scanning this week

☐  Diary of Reactive Habits

    ☐  First stressful situation

    ☐  Second stressful situation

# Interoceptive Awareness Indicator

Complete this after your first unilateral body scanning practice. Please color the parts in the silhouette where you can feel any type of body sensations. It's OK if you go slightly over the silhouette edge.

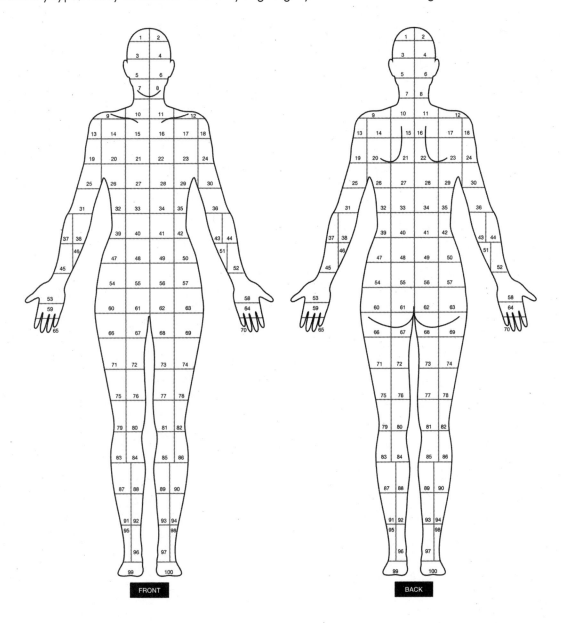

Total interoceptive awareness = _____% front + _____% back / 2 = _____%

## Interoceptive Awareness Indicator

Complete this after your most recent unilateral body scanning practice. Please color the parts in the silhouette where you can feel any type of body sensations. It's OK if you go slightly over the silhouette edge.

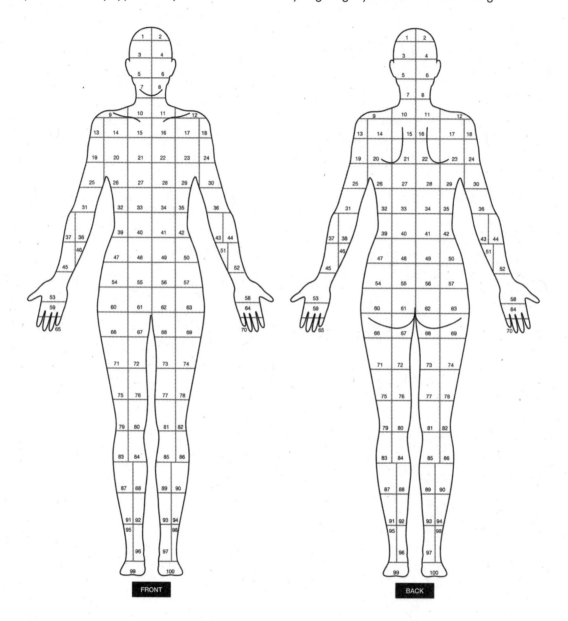

Total interoceptive awareness = _____% front + _____% back / 2 = _____%

## Daily Record of Unilateral Body Scanning Practice

| Day | Date | Morning Practice | Duration (Minutes) | Equanimity Rating<br><br>Rate from 1 to 10 how much equanimity you had while feeling body sensations.<br>1 = minimal; 10 = full | Evening Practice | Duration (Minutes) | Equanimity Rating<br><br>Rate from 1 to 10 how much equanimity you had while feeling body sensations.<br>1 = minimal; 10 = full |
|---|---|---|---|---|---|---|---|
| Day 1 | | yes / no | | | yes / no | | |
| Day 2 | | yes / no | | | yes / no | | |
| Day 3 | | yes / no | | | yes / no | | |
| Day 4 | | yes / no | | | yes / no | | |
| Day 5 | | yes / no | | | yes / no | | |
| Day 6 | | yes / no | | | yes / no | | |
| Day 7 | | yes / no | | | yes / no | | |

# Learning to Regulate Your Emotions

In week 4, we focus on incorporating equanimity into daily life. By applying equanimity to the four basic characteristics of body sensations, you can manage strong emotions skillfully. This approach will help you address challenging situations more effectively. We'll refine the practice of unilateral body scanning this week, by practicing in silence and without moving, to bolster equanimity training.

## Review of Last Week's Practices

Congratulations on completing your first week of body scanning! How did the week go? Were you able to maintain your commitment to practicing thirty minutes twice daily? Did you notice sensations in some parts of the body? Were you able to feel some intense sensations without reacting to them?

### What Did You Notice?

Here is a list of some of the experiences you may have had in your meditation practice. Check off the items that you noticed in at least some of your practices (and keep in mind that it is more important at this stage of the program to be aware of *what* you experience, rather than trying to have a certain *kind* of experience):

- ☐ Sensations in my body

- ☐ Thoughts in my mind

- ☐ Sensations in my body co-arising with thoughts in my mind

- ☐ Thoughts in my mind co-arising with sensations in my body

Which of these three kinds of sensations did you feel in the body? Check all that apply:

- ☐ Pleasant sensations

- ☐ Unpleasant sensations

- ☐ Neutral sensations

Although we are training equanimity, it is equally important to recognize when we are reacting! Which of the following did you experience during mindfulness practice this week? Check off all that apply:

- ☐ Reactivity to sensations
- ☐ Non-reactivity to sensations
- ☐ Wishing sensations were different
- ☐ Acceptance of sensations
- ☐ Trying to change sensations
- ☐ Welcoming sensations equanimously

If you practiced regularly during the week, it's likely that you experienced a decrease in reactivity by the end of the week. If it was a challenge to fit in enough practice sessions to begin developing these skills, it is important to acknowledge this without blaming yourself. Instead, we encourage you to be kind and patient with yourself, and recommit to your practice with a smile. Remember that being friendly towards yourself doesn't cost anything, and it can go a long way in helping you overcome any obstacles you may encounter.

If you are finding it difficult to feel sensations during practice, or are continually distracted by thoughts, it will be helpful to delay moving on to the next practice. We suggest returning to practicing mindfulness of breath a little more, until your mind settles, and you're more able to sustain focus on your breath. Then return to scanning the body with the audio instructions for a few days or even a full week, until you can feel at least twenty percent of the body surface.

Now, take a moment to look back at the two Interoceptive Awareness Indicator forms you completed last week, and jot down the numbers below. Did the percentage change between the first and last practice of the week?

| First Body Scanning Practice | Most Recent Body Scanning Practice |
|---|---|
| Date: | Date: |
| Percentage of body felt:          % | Percentage of body felt:          % |

We recommend proceeding to this week's body scanning practice when you can feel sensations over at least twenty percent of the body surface and are also able to hold back some craving and aversive reactions. For instance, feeling an itch and not scratching is an example of refraining from reacting out of aversion. Similarly, if you had a pleasant thought accompanied by pleasant sensations but continued to survey the body without allowing attention to linger on the pleasant sensations, you've successfully resisted reacting with craving.

Remember that it is normal to experience some intrusive thoughts, or areas of the body without much sensation. In fact, encountering these experiences with acceptance and an understanding of their imper-manence is an essential part of developing equanimity and insight. Therefore, don't wait to feel your entire body before starting to practice the next step, which is unilateral body scanning in silence—meaning, without listening to audio guidance.

## Unilateral Body Scanning in Silence

This week, you'll continue with the unilateral body scanning you were doing last week while progressing the practice in three ways: practicing in silence, increasing the scanning speed, and having the intention of refraining from moving while accepting your experience. By making these three changes, you'll be increasing the intensity of your practice and its effectiveness. Let's look at these practice refinements in more detail.

### Practicing in Silence

Practicing mindfulness with audio instructions is helpful when learning new skills, but it can also become a source of distraction and limit the efficiency of practice. After a week of practice, many people feel a growing need for silent practice.

There are several benefits to practicing body scanning in silence:

1. **Increased continuity of attention on body sensations:** When practicing in silence, attention does not need to shift back and forth between sensations and audio instructions. This sup-ports the development of more focused concentration.

2. **Following your own pace:** There is a lot of variation in how long it takes to develop the ability to consistently feel sensations in a particular area of the body. This is normal. It is helpful to move attention more slowly when you feel fewer or no sensations in a specific area, and practicing in silence this week allows you to do this.

3. **Desensitization of memories:** Because we are not adding the extra stimulus of the voice in the audio recording, we have more opportunities to observe spontaneously emerging thoughts, including memories, and their co-emerging body sensations with equanimity. When we choose to not react to the sensations, we gradually replace any previous reactivity associated with them with equanimity. In other words, these memories become less emotionally charged.

In essence, silent practice helps decondition the reactivity of our past, amplifying the already significant benefits of this kind of meditation practice.

## Practicing with Strong Determination

Completing difficult tasks in daily life requires determination. Without it, we might abandon our efforts when results aren't immediate. Practicing with "strong determination" in meditation involves making a strong commitment to develop equanimity during practice and one powerful way to cultivate equanimity is to commit to practicing in stillness.

Remaining very still during practice deepens our exploration of two key aspects of our experience. Firstly, committing to not move any part of the body offers the opportunity to observe habitual reactivity in the mind. We might find ourselves thinking *I must scratch that itch!* or *If I don't shift my position, I will scream!* We can observe craving and aversion arise in the mind in response to the simple act of sitting still while preventing conditioned reactions. These are valuable opportunities to experience unpleasant sensations with equanimity, choosing to feel them as they are, without harboring a hidden agenda to change them in any way.

Secondly, remaining very still allows us to observe the impermanence of all experiences, whether pleasant or unpleasant. When we move the body every time a sensation is unpleasant, we miss the opportunity to witness this fundamental reality. Remaining completely immobile allows you to observe unpleasant sensations without interruption and, after a short period of equanimous observation, to notice how the sensation and its intensity changes. This profound realization regarding impermanence is one of the most important understandings to develop in your practice. This insight is achievable because you are practicing exposure to the sensation rather than avoidance of it.

Make a strong commitment to sitting in stillness from here on out, and observe all experiences with equanimity as much as you can. When you do this, you are building skills to respond calmly and thoughtfully to similarly uncomfortable situations in daily life.

# Working with Strong Emotions

At first glance, it may seem that an emotion, such as fear or happiness, is a single experience. However, as we explored last week, emotions are actually made up of thoughts and bodily sensations and are often accompanied by a need to react. In fact, when we experience intense emotions, we tend to be more aware of the reactive impulse than the body sensations that preceded it.

These sensations have four basic characteristics: mass (ranging from very light to very heavy), motion (ranging from very still to very fast), temperature (ranging from very cold to very hot), and density (ranging from very tight or constricted to very loose or expanding).

These four characteristics of bodily sensations are the building blocks of our emotions and of all physical experiences. Just as the many flavors of international cuisines are created by five basic tastes (sweet, salty, sour, bitter, and savory), all the felt experiences in our body are created by various combinations of these four basic building blocks of sensation.

It can be helpful to visually record your experience of these characteristics, using the Mindfulness-based Interoceptive Signature Scale we'll provide in this chapter, when you feel any sort of stress or strong emotion. Each emotion has its own common pattern in the body. For example, feeling sad often comes with feeling heavy (mass) and cold (temperature), fear can come with constriction (density) and trembling or agitation (motion), and feeling joy often comes with feeling light (mass) and loose or radiating (density).

The example below is of Juan, who recorded the four characteristics after his experience of anger during a disagreement with his parents. He described feeling hot and feeling his heart race in his chest. Notice that temperature and motion were the most prominent characteristics for him in his experience. This is commonly the case with anger. You'll also note that the "Intensity After" measure is left incomplete. This scale relates to the mindfulness-based interoceptive exposure task, which we'll introduce you to in the next section.

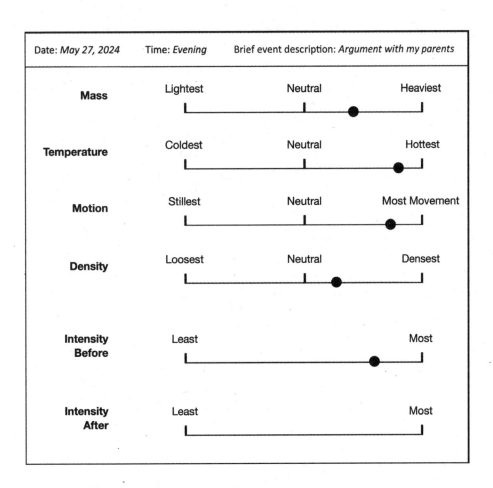

# Applying Your Skills: Approaching Strong Emotions with Equanimity

There are many opportunities to integrate the beneficial mindfulness skills you are learning into your daily life. This week we'll be focusing on bringing these skills to challenging situations you encounter during the day. We will be doing this in a very specific way—by being equanimous with the four characteristics of body sensations during times of emotional intensity, using the mindfulness-based interoceptive exposure task.

By using the four characteristics to focus on the sensory aspects of emotions, you'll be able to experience emotions more objectively, as you won't identify with them as much. While it is easy to take our sadness, fear, or anger personally, it is much harder to perceive temperature, mass, motion and density as part of who we are!

## Mindfulness-based Interoceptive Exposure Task (MIET)

The *mindfulness-based interoceptive exposure task* is a short, thirty-second applied mindfulness practice that you can use anytime, anywhere, to apply equanimity to your internal experience during stressful situations. This short practice guides you through the steps of feeling and identifying body sensations in terms of their four essential characteristics. Our research shows that observing mass, temperature, motion, and density with unconditional acceptance for thirty seconds can decrease associated distress and intensity by about fifty percent, including when the sensations are caused by chronic pain (Cayoun et al. 2020). The MIET will also form the foundation for applying mindfulness skills in stage 2, so your efforts this week will continue to benefit you and facilitate your progress over the next several weeks.

### Steps of the MIET

1.  When you experience a distressing event or challenging emotion, quickly scan the body to find the area of strongest sensations.

2.  Rate the intensity of sensations in this area by placing a small dot on the "Intensity Before" scale.

3.  Place a dot on each of the four other scales (mass, motion, temperature, and density) where it best represents the sensations you feel. For example, if the sensation feels very heavy, mark a small dot near the end of the "Mass" scale, close to "Heaviest."

4.  Draw a line joining the four dots. This is the "pre-equanimity line."

5.  Focus your attention on the four characteristics with equanimity for about half a minute. As a reminder, equanimity means approaching the sensations with a genuine willingness to feel them with acceptance, while preventing reactivity.

6.  After thirty seconds, place another dot on each of the four scales, representing how each of the characteristics feels after practicing equanimity.

7.  Join these dots with a dotted line. This is the "post-equanimity line."

8.  Record the change in intensity by placing a small dot on the "Intensity After" scale.

The difference between Intensity Before and Intensity After, as well as the distance between the dots of the pre-equanimity line and the post-equanimity line, shows the change that took place in your experience within thirty seconds.

Although each person has their own unique way of experiencing happiness, worry, hope, and so on, there are some common patterns that emerge. Studies have found that different emotions are associated with distinct patterns of bodily sensations, which are culturally universal (Nummenmaa et al. 2013). We have already seen the common pattern experienced with anger in Juan's example above.

In this next example, we return to Susan, whose story we discussed in chapter 2. When she first started practicing the MIET in week 4, she recognized that most of her experiences of sadness followed a pattern like in the example below. Notice that by allowing her attention to rest on the area of most intense sensations with a sense of curiosity, and a genuine willingness to experience and accept mass, motion, temperature, and density as they were in that moment, she was able to observe how the sensations changed over the thirty seconds. Note that this would not have happened if her intention during the practice had been to get rid of the unpleasant sensations.

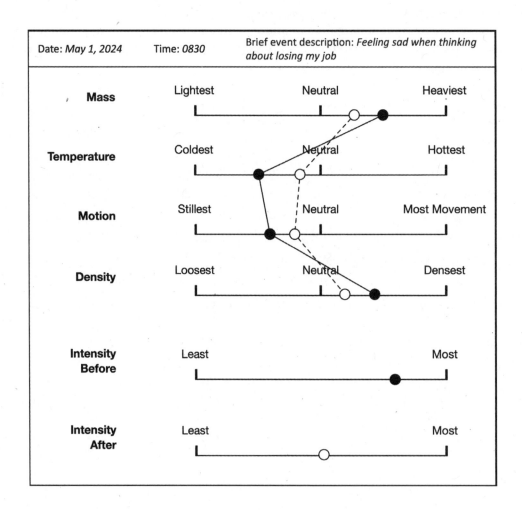

In this next example, Alex is a college student who has been juggling part time work with their studies. As midterms are approaching, Alex is feeling increasingly overwhelmed and anxious. Although there is a lot of variation in the experience of anxiety in the body, Alex's experience of feeling agitated (more movement), with cold hands (more cool) and constriction in the chest (more density) is common. As Alex focused on the area of most intense sensation in their hands, they experienced the four characteristics as follows:

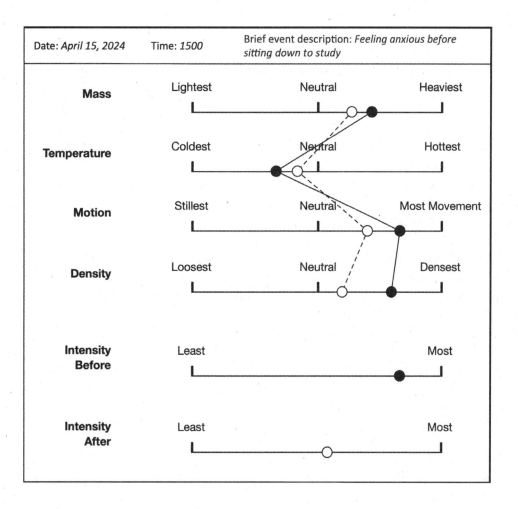

The above examples are of a single emotion. Often, we will find ourselves experiencing a mix of emotions, such as sadness and anger, or excitement and anxiety. In these cases, the dots won't follow the common patterns shown in the examples above, and instead will form their own particular combinations. This is to be expected. Your experience is unique to you, and your own patterns of single and mixed emotions will become apparent to you over time as you use the MIET.

# Practice Tips

Here are some tips to keep in mind as you begin your practice of the MIET:

## What if I forget to do the MIET during the stressful situation itself?

This is not a problem! It is still very valuable to go through the steps of the MIET as soon as possible afterward. You can think back to the intensity of initial distress, and this will help you feel some of the associated sensations again. Go through the steps of the MIET using these sensations, and then record the sensations, as well as their overall intensity, after completing the thirty-second exposure. Practicing in this way will help you learn the steps, and you will find that you can use this thirty-second practice more and more frequently during the stressful situations themselves.

## When I used the MIET, the intensity of distress increased after thirty seconds, instead of decreasing. Why did this happen?

This can occur for a few reasons. For example, if we had been avoiding feeling the unpleasant sensations, it can then take longer than thirty seconds to become fully aware of them. If this happens, not to worry: simply repeat another thirty-second exposure, focusing on the sensations with equanimity, without resisting in any way. Other times, the intensity of distress increases because we are still engaged to some degree in thinking about the situation, often about what it means to us. If this is the case, release attention from the thoughts, and refocus fully and equanimously on the characteristics of temperature, mass, motion, and density of the sensations.

Bringing equanimity to our moment-to-moment experience doesn't mean we are becoming indifferent or unresponsive to life's events. In fact, it's the opposite! We are allowing ourselves to both observe and fully feel our experience as it's unfolding. We become *more* connected to our experience, rather than disconnected from it. Our capacity to feel intense sensations with acceptance increases, whether the sensations are unpleasant or pleasant. We become more able to be present for both difficulty and joy, with an understanding that both arise and pass away. By developing our capacity to be with challenging emotions, we also expand our ability to experience positive, helpful ones.

## Egolessness

All sensations, pleasant, unpleasant, and neutral, are made of the same four characteristics, with some characteristics more apparent than others in any given situation. As we learn to perceive body sensations in terms of these characteristics, we are less likely to associate these sensations with a sense of self. Practicing the MIET regularly and recording the four characteristics visually is key, because it supports us in reappraising sensations in an impersonal way.

Through your practice, you'll develop insight into the impermanence of your thoughts, sensations, views, and attitudes, recognizing that they continually arise and pass, and don't determine who you are. You can learn to not attach to them, relating to them more lightly. In this way, you can break the cycle of suffering that would otherwise occur when things change in an unwanted direction.

## This Week's Practice

This week, refer to the practice instructions below to support your twice-daily unilateral body scanning. Use your Daily Record of Unilateral Body Scanning Practice in Silence to track your practice daily, and complete an Interoceptive Awareness Indicator after your last practice this week.

# Practice Instructions for Unilateral Body Scanning in Silence

- Practice in silence.

- Practice with strong determination: without moving and with unconditional acceptance.

- There will be some movements that arise spontaneously, such as coughing, sneezing, swallowing, and burping. These kinds of movements are generally not associated with attachment or aversion and can be allowed to unfold naturally. You are also welcome to straighten your posture if you are slouching.

- Remember to feel, accept, and move on. By being willing to feel sensations, we are less likely to react to them with aversion. By being willing to release attention from sensations and move on to the next area of the body, we are less likely to react to them with attachment.

- It is helpful to move attention more slowly when you feel fewer or no sensations in a specific area. There are many helpful changes in the brain taking place during this time, even if it feels like there is not a lot going on when you are focusing on a "blank spot"! And if you feel detailed sensations in some areas of the body, you can move attention through these areas more quickly, resulting in more cycles through the body. A "body cycle" consists of moving attention from the head to the toes and back to the head.

- Accelerate the speed of scanning, so that by the end of the week you are scanning two to three body cycles in thirty minutes. Going through more body cycles in each practice with equanimity increases the amount of exposure and opportunities for desensitization.

- If you find that you're readily distracted by thoughts and struggle to focus on sensations, start with ten minutes of mindfulness of breath practice and then move to twenty minutes of unilateral body scanning in silence. You may find it helpful to do this for several practice sessions before resuming thirty minutes of scanning practice.

- If you encounter a particularly intense sensation that repeatedly draws your attention, focus your attention at the center of the sensation with equanimity. Examine it closely without reacting to it. Study it while practicing the MIET. Focus on the predominant characteristics of the sensation, such as heaviness, constriction, heat, or movement. Remain calmly and patiently focused on it for about half a minute. If the intensity of the sensation decreases after this time, continue scanning the body. If the intensity persists, continue bringing attention to it with equanimity for up to two minutes before moving on.

Also remember to apply the thirty-second MIET practice as often as you can during the day. When first learning to implement the MIET, you can use audio track 11 to assist your practice. Record the results of your MIET practice on the record form. This will assist you in perceiving emotions more objectively in daily life. You can use the MIET forms provided in this workbook and print out additional copies, available online (http://www.newharbinger.com/52571). Recording your MIET practice multiple times will allow you to see patterns in how you experience emotions in your body.

You can compare ratings from the beginning of the week to the end of the week. Does the post-equanimity line get a little closer to the "Neutral" point as the week progresses? If so, this shows that when faced with a similar level of intensity, the amount of reactivity in your nervous system is decreasing.

---

## Week 4 Checklist

☐ Unilateral body scanning with strong determination: _____ /14

    ☐ Practice in silence, without audio instructions

    ☐ Daily Record of Unilateral Body Scanning Practice in Silence

☐ IAI worksheet at the end of week 4

☐ MIET

    ☐ Audio Track 11: use as a guide the first several times

    ☐ Record your MIET practice daily

## Daily Record of Unilateral Body Scanning Practice in Silence

| Day | Date | Morning Practice | Duration (Minutes) | Equanimity Rating Rate from 1 to 10 how much equanimity you had while feeling body sensations. 1 = minimal; 10 = full | Evening Practice | Duration (Minutes) | Equanimity Rating Rate from 1 to 10 how much equanimity you had while feeling body sensations. 1 = minimal; 10 = full |
|---|---|---|---|---|---|---|---|
| Day 1 | | yes / no | | | yes / no | | |
| Day 2 | | yes / no | | | yes / no | | |
| Day 3 | | yes / no | | | yes / no | | |
| Day 4 | | yes / no | | | yes / no | | |
| Day 5 | | yes / no | | | yes / no | | |
| Day 6 | | yes / no | | | yes / no | | |
| Day 7 | | yes / no | | | yes / no | | |

# Mindfulness-based Interoceptive Exposure Task (MIET)

## Instructions

When you experience a distressing event, notice the body sensations associated with it, both before and after, bringing equanimity to the sensations for thirty seconds. As soon as you can (either during the event itself, or shortly after), use one of the blank forms below to record your experience of body sensations in each of the four categories (mass, temperature, motion, density).

Start by placing a small dot on each of the four lines before applying equanimity, and join the dots with a line. This is the "pre-equanimity line." Then place another dot on each of the four categories to represent body sensations after practicing thirty seconds of full acceptance of sensations without reactivity. Then join those dots with a dotted line, the "post-equanimity line." Also record the change in intensity by placing small dots where appropriate on the "Intensity Before" and "Intensity After" lines.

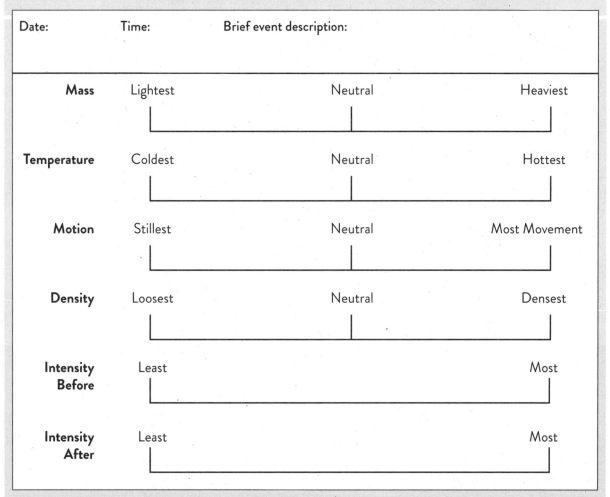

| Date: | Time: | Brief event description: | |
|---|---|---|---|

| | | | |
|---|---|---|---|
| **Mass** | Lightest | Neutral | Heaviest |
| **Temperature** | Coldest | Neutral | Hottest |
| **Motion** | Stillest | Neutral | Most Movement |
| **Density** | Loosest | Neutral | Densest |
| **Intensity Before** | Least | | Most |
| **Intensity After** | Least | | Most |

For additional copies of the MIET, visit http://www.newharbinger.com/52571.

## Interoceptive Awareness Indicator

Complete this after your first unilateral body scanning practice. Please color the parts in the silhouette where you can feel any type of body sensations. It's OK if you go slightly over the silhouette edge.

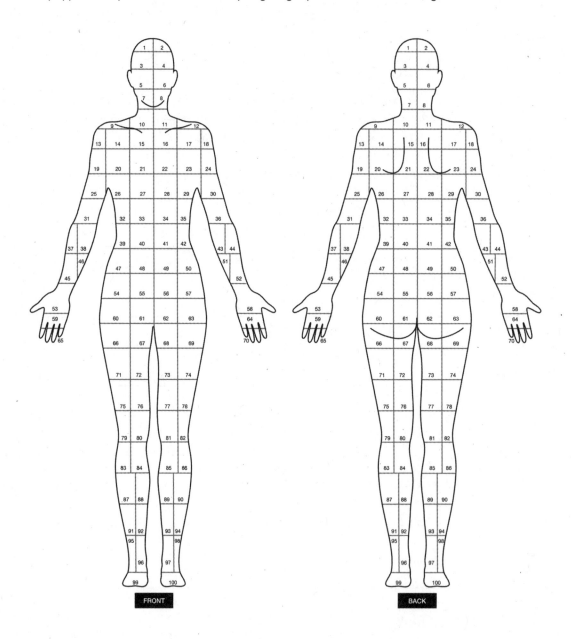

Total interoceptive awareness = _____% front + _____% back / 2 = _____%

*WEEK 5*

# Overcoming Avoidance

Week 5 marks the beginning of stage 2 of MiCBT, which focuses on using mindfulness skills to reduce habitual avoidance patterns that can reinforce anxiety and depression. This chapter delves into the mechanisms underlying avoidant behaviors, guiding you through exposure methods that combine visualization with equanimity towards body sensations. These techniques diminish fear and foster a greater sense of self-efficacy and confidence in taking healthy risks, such as socializing. During this week, you'll also learn a more advanced body scanning method, "symmetrical scanning," which further develops interoceptive awareness and equanimity—key tools for reducing avoidance.

## Review of Last Week's Practices

Congratulations on completing your second week of body scanning! Were you able to maintain your commitment to practicing thirty minutes twice daily? How was your practice with strong determination to remain immobile and equanimous? Were you able to prevent scratching an itch or not move when feeling restless? And how was your experience of using the MIET during stressful situations?

If you maintained a regular and accurate practice during the week, it is likely that you are now more able to sit in stillness and refrain from reacting, and consequently can feel sensations in more parts of the body. If it was difficult to practice regularly, it's important to acknowledge this without blaming yourself. Instead of judging yourself, we encourage you to be kind towards yourself and recommit to your practice with more confidence. Being able to change your attitude toward yourself is a great skill in itself.

Sometimes circumstances such as sleep deprivation, illness, or an increase in stressors can reduce our ability to focus on the body and make it harder to feel sensations. If this is the case for you, it can be helpful to return to practicing mindfulness of breath in silence for several days to regain your focus before moving on to symmetrical scanning, outlined below.

## Estimating Neuroplasticity

As before, take a moment to look back at the Interoceptive Awareness Indicator (IAI) to see the percentage of the body you could feel in your most recent body scanning practices, and jot down the number below. Could you feel more of the body this week than you could last week?

| Most Recent Practice |
| --- |
| Date: |
| Percentage of body felt:                  % |

## Reviewing Interoceptive Signatures

How did it go with practicing the MIET during day-to-day challenging situations? Could you remain objective with emotions? Do you notice at times that the emotions you feel are made up of the characteristics of mass, motion, temperature, and density, rather than being parts of who you are? If you recorded at least seven MIET practices in the past week, you may already be seeing your own unique patterns in the four characteristics with different emotions. With regular MIET practice, it will become increasingly easier to feel the very beginning of challenging emotions, accept the experience without identifying with it, and let it pass without having to react.

# Symmetrical Scanning

This week, you'll start practicing a more advanced body-scanning technique, called symmetrical scanning. Each technique we learn along the MiCBT journey is beneficial in its own right, and is also a stepping stone for the next practice. As such, symmetrical scanning lays the foundation for the method you'll be learning next week.

In *symmetrical scanning*, attention is directed part by part towards both sides of the body at the same time. For example, rather than directing your attention to first one cheek and then the other, you focus attention on both cheeks at the same time.

Because the brain is connected slightly differently in each hemisphere, as you move attention down both sides of the body simultaneously, you may feel more sensations on one side of the body in certain areas than in the others. For instance, while you might initially feel the left side of the scalp more easily than the right, the right forearm might be more perceptible than the left. Many of these differences will subside over time.

When first starting to practice, you may also notice that your attention moves from one side of the body first, then the other. This "lead-lag" is completely normal and after a few days of zigzagging rapidly across both sides of the body, you'll be able to scan both sides symmetrically, "in-phase."

## Specific Benefits

Progressing to symmetrical scanning results in an increase in the number of times that attention is passed through the body in a thirty-minute practice. The benefits of this include:

1. **Increasing desensitization.** Surveying sensations throughout the body equanimously a greater number of times during the same practice session accelerates the desensitization process. This, in turn, reduces both the frequency and intensity of learned reactivity.

2. **Enhanced neuroplasticity.** Increasing the number of scans through parts of the body where it is difficult to feel sensations increases the frequency with which neurons connect to allow us to feel sensation in those areas. By increasing these brain connections, especially in the areas of the somatosensory cortex and insular cortex—key areas of the brain for processing body sensations—we become progressively able to feel body sensations clearly in areas that were initially "blank" or unclear.

3. **Setting the stage for partial sweeping.** Symmetrical scanning is also a pre-requisite skill for the next advanced method, partial sweeping, which will be introduced next week, as it serves as a stepping stone to rapidly feeling detailed sensations in more and more areas of the body.

## The Nature of Avoidance

Avoidance itself is neither good nor bad. In some circumstances, it is an adaptive way of protecting ourselves from harm, as it can steer us away from danger, pain, loss, and failure. However, it can also become problematic and significantly limit our lives. Maladaptive avoidance is common in depression and anxiety, and can deprive us of beneficial experiences, including activities we cherish and wish to take part in.

When anxious or depressed, we tend to avoid socializing, spending time with family, or being intimate with a partner, all of which can contribute to a sense of isolation and loneliness. Over time, this can worsen symptoms. Maladaptive avoidance also often includes avoiding taking healthy risks, which over time can contribute to a lack of self-confidence. These are just a few examples of how avoidant behavior can maintain symptoms of depression and anxiety, which makes addressing avoidant behavior a key part of treatment.

## What Are We Really Avoiding?

When avoiding situations which you believe will make you feel stressed, depressed, or anxious, what are you really avoiding? It may be helpful to revisit the co-emergence model of reinforcement discussed in chapter 3, as it is very relevant here. Every time we anticipate that a situation will create anxiety, even just the thought of it can create co-emerging unpleasant sensations in the body.

If we don't recognize this pattern, we might believe that it's the situation itself which makes us feel anxious, which can lead to avoiding the situation altogether. The accompanying feeling of relief reinforces the belief that avoidance is helpful. This belief is reinforced every time we avoid the situation again, and we remain unaware that what we are *actually* avoiding are the unpleasant body sensations that make up the experience of anxiety.

For this reason, overcoming avoidance requires desensitizing to unpleasant sensations in situations that you would typically avoid. The skills you have developed so far will be extremely valuable. Since you have already started to be more equanimous with unpleasant body sensations, all you need to do is to apply equanimity in situations you no longer wish to avoid. In MiCBT, we use evidence-based exposure methods to decrease the discomfort that comes with exposure and reduce anxiety. Let's start!

## Preparing for Exposure

Begin by creating a list of ten to twelve activities and situations that you would benefit from no longer avoiding. Let's call them "items." Once you have written them down in the table below, write down the percentage of distress you believe they would cause you if you were to go and do them right now. A 0% means not distressing at all, and 100% means the greatest level of distress, such as a very severe panic attack. For example, if you have moderately severe social anxiety and you avoid being around people you don't know, then your rated item could be: "Being around strangers: 60%."

Try to vary the items in your list. It's best if they are not all related to the same fear, so that your confidence in preventing avoidance will *generalize* to many aspects of your life—that is, carry over into other situations—rather than being limited to a specific context. For example, if you have symptoms of claustrophobia, only include up to two items related to your avoidance of confined spaces, and include items related to other situations. Also, we're only brainstorming at this stage, so write down all the items that come to mind; you'll be able to select specific ones from this list later.

Below is an example of brainstormed items, each rated with a percentage of distress:

- Changing to a healthier diet: 60%

- Being around big dogs without muzzles in public spaces: 25%

- Going to the gym: 40%

- Going to the dentist: 55%

- Wearing colorful clothes: 70%

- Speaking in public: 90%

- Being outside late at night: 15%

- Looking for a job: 45%

- Speaking to my partner about our issues: 100%

- Telling my boss I want to work part-time beginning next year: 80%

- Not drinking alcohol in the evening: 35%

- Reconnecting with my sister: 70%

Now it's your turn. Complete the Avoided Situation or Activity table below and the SUDS (Subjective Units of Distress Scale) Sheet today, as you'll be starting your first bipolar exposure to SUDS item one this evening if possible. Remember, integrating bipolar exposure adds eleven to twelve minutes, so you'll need to adjust your routines accordingly, knowing that your efforts will yield substantial benefits!

| Avoided Situation or Activity | Distress Rating (%) |
| --- | --- |
| | |
| | |
| | |
| | |
| | |
| | |
| | |
| | |
| | |
| | |
| | |
| | |

Once you have a list of ten to twelve avoided items and have rated each with a distress score, it's time to select the ones you'll use for your exposure practice.

## Subjective Units of Distress Scale Item List

Select five items from your brainstormed list that range from low to high levels of distress. The lowest intensity item should create between twenty and thirty percent distress. Items below twenty percent distress generally don't create as many unpleasant sensations, so they are not very useful for our purposes.

On the other hand, having a first item that causes more than about 30 percent distress may be too daunting to start with. Therefore, to ensure that you feel confident starting the first exposure task, your first item should create some unpleasant sensations but also be readily achievable.

Here is an example of five items selected from the list above:

| SUDS Sheet | Day 1 | | Day 7 | | Day 14 | |
|---|---|---|---|---|---|---|
| Situation or Activity | Date | Distress Rating | Date | Distress Rating | Date | Distress Rating |
| Being around big dogs without muzzles in public spaces | Nov 19 | 25% | | | | |
| Going to the gym | Nov 19 | 40% | | | | |
| Going to the dentist | Nov 19 | 55% | | | | |
| Wearing colorful clothes | Nov 19 | 70% | | | | |
| Speaking in public | Nov 19 | 90% | | | | |

Fill in the first three columns of the SUDS table below, listing your items along with today's date and distress ratings. The last four columns will be used to record distress ratings next week (Day 7), and the following week (Day 14).

| SUDS Sheet | Day 1 | | Day 7 | | Day 14 | |
|---|---|---|---|---|---|---|
| Situation or Activity | Date | Distress Rating | Date | Distress Rating | Date | Distress Rating |
| | | | | | | |
| | | | | | | |
| | | | | | | |
| | | | | | | |
| | | | | | | |

Now that you have a hierarchy of situations in place, we can turn to the kind of exposures you'll be doing. The first exposure method, called bipolar exposure, is done using your imagination, and the second, *in vivo* exposure, is done in real life.

## Applying Your Skills: Equanimity During Exposure

One advantage of starting exposure using imagery is that you can practice facing the avoided situation while feeling safe and not overly distressed. Another advantage is that you are in control of the process and can interrupt it at any time. Once you've done sufficient exposure using imagery, you'll be ready and more confident to use your skills in real life situations. And once anxiety in certain situations has been clearly understood as a fear of feeling particular body sensations, exposure to the feared situation in real life rapidly becomes productive and rewarding. When we have less "fear of fear in the body," we develop a new sense of confidence and empowerment.

# The Bipolar Exposure Method

*Bipolar exposure* uses visualization to expose to two opposite "poles" of the same situation, one unpleasant and the other pleasant, while remaining equanimous with body sensations that co-emerge during the imagined scenarios. Bipolar exposure is practiced right after your thirty-minute meditation practice. You'll be practicing bipolar exposure with your first SUDS item four times before exposing yourself to the situation in real life.

Here are the steps of bipolar exposure, using the 25% distress example of being in a park close to a large dog:

1.  Just after finishing body scanning, while remaining seated, open your eyes to start playing track 15, the guided instructions to practice bipolar exposure, which is eleven minutes long. After closing your eyes again, begin imagining the worst things that could happen two days from now, when you are around the dog in real life. Apply your equanimity to any sensations that arise while catastrophizing the event; you may need several "worst-case" scenarios for the five minutes. Remind yourself that sensations are made of four characteristics (mass, motion, temperature, and density) that just arise to pass away. They are in a continual state of change, and there is no need to react to get rid of them.

2.  After five minutes of exposure to unpleasant sensations, rest your mind on your breath, focusing at the entrance of the nostrils while breathing calmly and peacefully for about a minute or a little longer if it is needed for your mind and breath to settle. Keep at the back of your mind that all this is only occurring in the imagination, and you are in full control throughout the entire exercise.

3.  Then restart imagining being around the dog two days from now, but this time imagine the best-case scenarios for five minutes. Embellish them as much as possible while keeping the story realistic. This time, the co-emerging sensations will be pleasant, though it's not always easy to feel pleasant sensations on the first or second attempt. This is because the brain is evolutionarily predisposed to produce experiences of unpleasant sensations more readily than pleasant ones.

4.  With practice, you are likely to start feeling pleasant sensations more easily by your third or fourth imaginal exposure. Do your best to not become attached to feeling these pleasant sensations. This will help prevent being dissatisfied if you don't feel pleasant sensations when you are around the animal in real life.

5.  Once you have practiced bipolar exposure four times using item 1, start with real life expo-sure. At the same time, begin bipolar exposure with item 2 (e.g., "going to the gym" in our previous example) for the next two days while doing *in vivo* exposure to item 1. Follow the same process for all five items.

---

30 minutes practicing body scanning

⇩

5 minutes visualizing worst case scenarios with equanimity

⇩

1 to 2 minutes practicing mindfulness of breath

⇩

5 minutes visualizing best case scenarios with equanimity

---

To support your practice of bipolar exposure, you might take some time now to write down the first situation you'll be practicing with and some of the worst- and best-case scenarios for it.

Situation 1: _____

_____

_____

Worst-case scenarios: _____

_____

_____

_____

Best-case scenarios: _____

_____

_____

_____

Over the next two weeks, you'll be continuing to increase your equanimity using this safe approach to expose yourself to more and more intense body sensations.

## The In Vivo Exposure Method

Despite the benefits of bipolar exposure alone, exposure to real life situations—or in vivo *exposure*—is important and necessary to change unhelpful habits (Boettcher and Barlow 2019). *In vivo* is a Latin phrase used by therapists to describe exposure in real life.

When you go into the situation in real life, the most important thing to remember is to remain equanimous. This is a training in exposure to sensations with equanimity—each time you complete a SUDS item in daily life is one more valuable opportunity to feel unpleasant sensations without reactivity and without making it be about you. This is one of the most effective ways to train equanimity.

Here is a summary of daily exposure activities this week. We will continue with a similar exposure structure with the last two items on your list next week.

| Day 1 and Day 2 | Day 3 and Day 4 | Day 5 to Day 7 |
|---|---|---|
| Bipolar exposure to item 1 | Bipolar exposure to item 2<br><br>+<br><br>Daily *in vivo* exposure to item 1 | Bipolar exposure to item 3<br><br>+<br><br>Daily *in vivo* exposure to items 1 and 2 |

You can also use the following tracking tool to stay on track with your exposure practice, if you find it helpful.

We have completed the first table using SUDS items from Susan, whom you met in chapter 2. You can see that on Day 5 she will be completing *in vivo* exposure to SUDS items one and two, and starting bipolar exposure to her third SUDS item, "calling a friend."

| Exposure Tracking Tool (Example) | Bipolar Exposure to Item 1 | Bipolar Exposure to Item 2 | Daily In Vivo Exposure to Items 1 and 2 | Bipolar Exposure to Item 3 | Daily In Vivo Exposure to Item 3 |
|---|---|---|---|---|---|
| Day 1 | Exercising | | | | |
| Day 2 | Exercising | | | | |
| Day 3 | | Shopping in town | Exercising | | |
| Day 4 | | Shopping in town | Exercising | | |
| Day 5 | | | Exercising and shopping in town | Calling a friend | |
| Day 6 | | | Exercising and shopping in town | Calling a friend | |
| Day 7 | | | Exercising and shopping in town | | Calling a friend |

The second table is for you to write in your exposure items.

| Exposure Tracking Tool | Bipolar Exposure to Item 1 | Bipolar Exposure to Item 2 | Daily In Vivo Exposure to Items 1 and 2 | Bipolar Exposure to Item 3 | Daily In Vivo Exposure to Item 3 |
|---|---|---|---|---|---|
| Day 1 | | | | | |
| Day 2 | | | | | |
| Day 3 | | | | | |
| Day 4 | | | | | |
| Day 5 | | | | | |
| Day 6 | | | | | |
| Day 7 | | | | | |

## This Week's Practice

As in previous weeks, you can track your practice of symmetrical scanning using the Daily Record form that follows. Use audio tracks 12 and 13 for your first two practices, and then just audio track 13 with each of the practices that follow.

Do your best to follow the bipolar and *in vivo* exposure schedule, but if you miss an exposure, it's important that you don't feel disheartened, and instead remain patient with yourself. Just resume your exposure as soon as possible, keeping in mind that equanimity needs to become increasingly part of your life, even when you can't immediately achieve what you want.

---

### Week 5 Checklist

☐ Symmetrical body scanning: _____ /14

    ☐ Audio Track 12: listen for the first two practices only

    ☐ Audio Track 13: listen with each practice

    ☐ Daily Record of Symmetrical Body Scanning Practice

☐ Fill out the Avoided Situation or Activity Table with up to twelve items

☐ Fill out the SUDS Sheet with five items for exposure, with initial date and distress rating

☐ Bipolar exposure and *in vivo* exposure to SUDS items 1, 2, and 3

    ☐ Audio Track 14: listen for the first two practices only

    ☐ Audio Track 15: listen with each practice

## Daily Record of Symmetrical Body Scanning Practice

| Day | Date | Morning Practice | Duration (Minutes) | Equanimity Rating Rate from 1 to 10 how much equanimity you had while feeling body sensations. 1 = minimal; 10 = full | Evening Practice | Duration (Minutes) | Equanimity Rating Rate from 1 to 10 how much equanimity you had while feeling body sensations. 1 = minimal; 10 = full |
|---|---|---|---|---|---|---|---|
| Day 1 | | yes / no | | | yes / no | | |
| Day 2 | | yes / no | | | yes / no | | |
| Day 3 | | yes / no | | | yes / no | | |
| Day 4 | | yes / no | | | yes / no | | |
| Day 5 | | yes / no | | | yes / no | | |
| Day 6 | | yes / no | | | yes / no | | |
| Day 7 | | yes / no | | | yes / no | | |

# WEEK 6

# Improving Self-Confidence

This week, we dive deeper into the exposure skills you started practicing last week, which are instrumental in reducing avoidance and fostering a newfound sense of self-confidence in your daily life. One powerful concept we'll explore is generalization of desensitization, and how you can use it to work in your favor. The next body scanning method, partial sweeping, focuses on developing interoceptive awareness of subtle and often pleasant body sensations. You'll also review your progress with exposure before progressing to the last two items on your list, using unpleasant sensations as tools for desensitization and cultivating a more equanimous mind.

## Review of Last Week's Practices

You have now completed your third week of body scanning, using the symmetrical scanning practice. Were you able to sometimes feel sensations on both sides of the body simultaneously? At the beginning of the week, it can initially feel like attention is moving from one side of the body to the other, but with regular practice, you might have found it easier to move your attention symmetrically down both sides of the body simultaneously.

When you can consistently feel around eighty percent of the body, even if not entirely symmetrically, you're ready to advance to partial sweeping. If you are not feeling close to eighty percent yet, continue practicing symmetrical scanning, in silence, for a few more days.

## Partial Sweeping

During *partial sweeping*, attention is moved continuously through large areas of the body, rather than moving part by part. Partial sweeping provides opportunities for developing equanimity towards both pleasant and unpleasant sensations, which is key for emotion regulation, as we'll see below.

## Practice Instructions

Begin with all of your attention at the top of your head and move your attention in a continuous fashion—"sweeping"—down to your neck, feeling sensations in as much of the scalp and face as you can. Once complete, continue to move attention slowly in a continuous sweeping motion vertically across your neck and throat, then both shoulders, arms, hands, and lastly, your fingertips.

Once the upper limbs are scanned, start with the torso. For the large area of the torso, it is best to start by dividing it into smaller parts. For the first two days, start with the entire front of the torso, moving downward from the base of your throat to the groin. Then, starting at the base of the neck, sweep your attention down the back to the buttocks. Then sweep both sides of the torso symmetrically, beginning from the armpits, down your sides to the hips. On the third day, do your best to combine the front and back of the torso simultaneously. From the fifth day onward, combine the front, back and sides of the torso in a single continual movement of attention. After the torso is scanned, continue to pass your attention symmetrically down the hips and buttocks area, and then down the legs and feet in a sweeping fashion. Once you reach the tips of the toes, slowly sweep back upward to the top of the head.

It's okay if you are not able to feel sensations in some areas at first. Sweep your attention through the body without interruption while noting these blank or unclear areas, and after two or three cycles, come back to these parts and survey them separately before resuming partial sweeping again. Keep scanning the body equanimously as many times as possible within your thirty-minute practice.

## Benefits of Feeling Subtle Body Sensations

As you refine your partial sweeping practice, you may begin to notice increasingly subtle sensations, some of which may feel quite pleasant. Experiencing these pleasant sensations is a result of increased connections between neurons and is one of several ways that the body scanning practice this week results in improved emotion regulation.

Firstly, subtle pleasant sensations are usually harder to feel than unpleasant sensations—and practicing feeling them during body scanning will help you feel them more readily in daily life. As we discussed in chapter 3, with depression and anxiety, it is difficult to feel sensations in the body, especially pleasant ones, yet we need to be able to feel pleasant sensations in order to enjoy our life! Learning to feel subtle pleasant sensations during body scanning will generalize to more readily being able to experience joy in daily life.

Another big benefit is that you'll be able to feel subtle unpleasant sensations sooner than before. How can this be good news? The reason is that these more subtle unpleasant sensations can serve as an early alert system, sending advance notice of potential distress before full-blown challenging emotions take form. This can give us the extra few seconds we need to pause before reacting and choose a more skillful way to go forward.

Finally, because partial sweeping involves moving attention through large parts of the body quickly, the waves of sensations we feel as a result can evoke wave-like emotions, and occasionally remind us of instances of joy, anger, or sadness, through the process of co-emergence. Sometimes we are not consciously aware of a specific emotion during practice—we might just feel a passing flush of heat or movement. Nonetheless, when we bring equanimity to these experiences, reactivity is neutralized, and we reap the benefits in daily life in the form of decreased reactivity to unhelpful emotions.

# The Nature of Attachment

Attachment can manifest in various forms, such as attachment to people, ideas, possessions, experiences, outcomes, our body, reputation, and sense of self. There are also healthy forms of attachment that form the foundation of our human relationships, which is not the kind of attachment we are referring to. Unhelpful attachment is a clinging onto experience, and is driven by craving, an age-old trap that tricks us into believing that what we crave will bring lasting satisfaction. We assign a special value and meaning to what we crave. But everything in life is transient, including the things we desire most, like pleasure and love. Ultimately, because of the unavoidable reality of impermanence, the consequence of attachment is grief. The stronger the attachment, the more intense the grief that follows loss will be.

## Attachment to Sensations

During mindfulness meditation practice, sensations arise and pass away, reminding us of the impermanence of experiences. However, the mind tends to react differently to these sensations based on whether they are perceived as unpleasant, pleasant, or neutral. We may crave pleasant sensations, resist unpleasant ones, and disregard neutral ones, all of which falls under the umbrella of attachment to having things be a certain way. Whether sensations bring memories of past pleasures or pains, our task is to observe them without clinging or rejecting, and without identifying them as "ours."

As your mindfulness practice deepens, you may discover subtle attachments that were previously overlooked, such as attachment to the pleasant flow of small tingling sensations during meditation, or even to the state of calm itself. Remember, if you become attached to these experiences, how will you feel when they are absent?

## Effect of Attachment on Mood and Anxiety

Attachment often leads to unrealistic expectations and standards, which, when unmet, cause stress, anxiety, and negative mood shifts. For instance, an attachment to being the best in every endeavor could create a high level of anxiety and contribute to a sense of failure in circumstances when being the best is not possible. Moreover, the attachment to pleasant experiences could create dissatisfaction and anxiety when those experiences change or cease.

While attachments can provide a temporary sense of comfort or identity, they can also serve as a major source of suffering due to their inherently impermanent nature. Recognizing impermanence can lead to a decrease in craving and aversion, and subsequently, to a decrease in suffering. Through practicing equanimity, we feel freer from attachment and begin to experience a more profound sense of calm and well-being.

# Applying Your Skills: Continuing Bipolar and In Vivo Exposure

How did it go with bipolar exposure? Were you able to feel unpleasant sensations when imagining the worst-case scenarios and pleasant sensations when imagining the best-case scenarios? Sometimes it can be more difficult to feel pleasant sensations than unpleasant ones! This is partly because of our emotional habits—we tend to practice feeling unpleasant sensations much more often than pleasant ones—and partly due to an evolutionary configuration of the brain.

After one week of practicing imaginal and *in vivo* exposure with SUDS items 1, 2, and 3, it is time to re-rate your distress levels associated with all five SUDS items. Turn to your SUDS Sheet in week 5 under Day 7 and fill in today's date and ratings for all five SUDS items, as it would feel if you were to go out now and do the *in vivo* (real life) exposure to the sensations that arise in these situations. Also do this for SUDS items 4 and 5, even though you have probably not started imaginal and *in vivo* exposures for these yet.

What do you notice? Is there a reduction in distress scores for SUDS items 1, 2, and 3? Perhaps some of these scores have started to decrease. If it is possible to keep exposing to items 1, 2, and 3 in real life, keep doing the *in vivo* exposures daily or as frequently as you can until the distress rating for these items is consistently around 5 to 10%.

And how about distress ratings for items 4 and 5? You may have experienced a decrease in distress ratings for these items, even though you have not yet done bipolar or *in vivo* exposure for them. This occurs because our increased confidence in feeling and managing anxiety-related body sensations in some situations generalizes to other situations in which we feel the same or similar anxiety sensations.

## Generalizing the Effects of Exposure

As discussed previously, prolonged avoidant behaviors can generalize to avoidance of other stressful situations. However, the power of generalization can also be harnessed to our advantage—reduction in avoidance and anxiety can generalize across similar situations. For example, if exposure to fear sensations with equanimity leads to reduced anxiety when meeting new people at a party, it is likely that anxiety when meeting new coworkers will also decrease.

We can also generalize our equanimity and decreased avoidance across situations that are different from each other. If you have been equanimous with sensations of anxiety when speaking in public, in addition to being less anxious about other social performances, you are also likely to be less anxious with other avoided situations, such as being close to a spider, walking on a bridge, being alcohol free on the weekend, or learning complicated skills, as the underlying sensations of anxiety are the same in these situations.

In all these scenarios, we are desensitizing to the unpleasant co-emerging sensations, rather than to the situations themselves. By recognizing the co-emerging sensations and feeling them with equanimity, we learn to manage anxiety effectively in a wide range of avoided situations.

Take the story of Chen, a young man who struggled with social anxiety, which led him to avoid interacting with others. After several weeks of practicing MiCBT, he started using exposure exercises to target anxiety-provoking situations, like attending parties or events. To his surprise, he noticed that his fear of heights, which was unrelated to his social anxiety, also started to diminish.

Why did this happen? As he became more skilled in bringing equanimity to the four characteristics of co-emerging sensations during social situations, his nervous system began generalizing equanimity towards sensations co-emerging with anxiety to other areas, including his fear of heights. His equanimity during exposure to one high-arousal state (social anxiety) led to a generalization of equanimity to another high-arousal state (fear of heights). He was unknowingly neutralizing his fear of heights without having to expose to heights themselves.

By desensitizing the unpleasant sensations associated with fear during exposure, you are actually deconditioning all fear reactions, across a wide range of situations, including those which may contribute to anxiety and depression.

## Adjusting SUDS Items 4 and 5

Take a moment to look at your SUDS 4 and 5 items in week 5. Double check that it will be possible to implement them in daily life this coming week. If not, choose other items with a similar level of distress intensity that you *can* implement this week. If item 4 involved presenting a five-minute project summary at a monthly progress meeting, creating 75% distress, but the meeting had been rescheduled until the following week, find another situation which you expect will also create roughly 75% distress and is possible to implement this next week.

## This Week's Practice

When practicing partial sweeping this week, remember to apply equanimity toward all sensations, even subtle and pleasant ones. Learning to remain equanimous and reduce attachment to pleasant sensations will reduce the habit of craving pleasant experiences in daily life and allow you to feel more at ease with sensations experienced in the present. Importantly, you may start to recognize similarities between sensations experienced during your meditation practice and those that arise in the body during the day.

Practice bipolar exposure to item 4 today and tomorrow, while continuing *in vivo* exposure to item 3, and on Day 3 this week, add *in vivo* exposure to item 4, while starting bipolar exposure to SUDS item 5 twice daily. Begin *in vivo* exposure to item 5 on Day 5.

| Day 1 and Day 2 | Day 3 and Day 4 | Day 5 to Day 7 |
|---|---|---|
| Bipolar exposure to item 4<br><br>+<br><br>Daily *in vivo* exposure to item 3 | Bipolar exposure to item 5<br><br>+<br><br>Daily *in vivo* exposure to items 3 and 4 | Daily *in vivo* exposure to items 4 and 5 |

As very challenging situations can require a little longer to address, it is OK if exposure to items 4 and 5 takes one or two additional days.

---

## Week 6 Checklist

☐ Partial sweeping: _____ /14

    ☐ Audio Track 16: for the first two practices only

    ☐ Audio Track 17: listen with each practice

    ☐ Daily Record of Partial Sweeping Practice

☐ Complete distress ratings on the SUDS Sheet at the beginning of this week, with today's date

☐ Bipolar exposure and *in vivo* exposure to SUDS items 4 and 5

## Daily Record of Partial Sweeping Practice

| Day | Date | Morning Practice | Duration (Minutes) | Equanimity Rating<br>Rate from 1 to 10 how much equanimity you had while feeling body sensations.<br>1 = minimal; 10 = full | Evening Practice | Duration (Minutes) | Equanimity Rating<br>Rate from 1 to 10 how much equanimity you had while feeling body sensations.<br>1 = minimal; 10 = full |
|---|---|---|---|---|---|---|---|
| Day 1 | | yes / no | | | yes / no | | |
| Day 2 | | yes / no | | | yes / no | | |
| Day 3 | | yes / no | | | yes / no | | |
| Day 4 | | yes / no | | | yes / no | | |
| Day 5 | | yes / no | | | yes / no | | |
| Day 6 | | yes / no | | | yes / no | | |
| Day 7 | | yes / no | | | yes / no | | |

# WEEK 7

# Bringing Mindfulness to Relationships

Welcome to week 7 of your MiCBT journey, a pivotal week where we apply mindfulness skills to interpersonal relationships. You will practice "sweeping *en masse*" to build on the mindfulness skills you've been developing over the past six weeks and apply them to understanding the emotions and reactions of others. Using the applied practice of "experiential ownership" will allow you to engage with others empathically, even in challenging interactions, without succumbing to reactivity. Get ready for another transformative week!

## Review of Last Week's Practices

Reflecting on the past week's body scanning practice of partial sweeping, could you move your attention through whole parts of the body in a single movement? Did you notice any areas of subtle, perhaps pleasant, sensations? These can sometimes feel like subtle tingly, electric sensations or vibrations.

At this stage, you may be able to feel subtle, distinct sensations throughout most of your body, with sensations in the limbs typically being more perceptible than in the torso. Being able to feel about eighty percent of the surface of the body over the course of a thirty-minute practice session means that you have enough interoceptive awareness and equanimity towards body sensations to move on to sweeping *en masse*. If you can't quite feel this eighty percent yet, take a few more days to continue practicing partial sweeping before moving on to sweeping *en masse*. In your brain's insular cortex, the increased connections between neurons that will result from this extra effort will be really beneficial when you start sweeping *en masse* a few days from now.

### Exposure to Avoided Situations

Were you able to complete exposure to SUDS items 4 and 5? If so, congratulations! This is a big achievement. You are ready to move on to exposure to interpersonal situations. If logistics got in the way, take a few more days to complete SUDS items 4 and 5—you'll be building on the equanimity that you develop during these exposures during the interpersonal exposures in week 7. Either way, remember to complete the chart in week 5 under Day 14 with today's date and ratings for all five SUDS items.

# Sweeping en Masse

*Sweeping en masse* is the next advanced body-scanning practice, and requires moving through the entire body in a continuous flow of attention, from the top of the head to the tips of the toes, and back again. It allows us to feel increasingly more body parts at the same time and even more subtle sensations with equanimity, whether unpleasant, pleasant, or neutral.

## Practice Instructions

Begin your practice of sweeping *en masse* with an uninterrupted movement of attention from the top of your head down the body vertically until you reach the tip of the toes and back up again, cycling down and up over the body continuously. You may need to move attention slowly at first, but by the end of the week, your attention will be flowing more smoothly and quickly.

When you encounter blank spots or areas where you can't feel sensations clearly, just as you did last week, note these areas without interrupting the flow of attention. After two or three cycles of sweeping, you may start to feel sensations in some of these areas. For the spots that have remained blank, go back and scan each one separately, using 2- to 3-inch areas. Things may seem not to change, at least not immediately; remain patient and equanimous, dedicating up to half a minute for each blank spot. Then go back to sweeping *en masse* for another two or three cycles, before returning to blank spots, further developing your equanimity.

Learning to remain equanimous with the absence of sensations also teaches you to remain equanimous when you can't get what you want in daily life. This is because we use the same brain in both the internal and external contexts of our lives. The attitude you have toward your experiences during meditation is the attitude you have in daily life. Therefore, noticing with equanimity that you are not experiencing what you would like while scanning the body is a great opportunity to transfer this skill into daily life, and remain patient and tolerant when your expectations are not met.

## Neutralizing Deep-Seated Emotions

With sweeping *en masse*, it is very normal and expected for there to be more intrusive thoughts. Because of this, you might notice that it is harder to stay focused on the body! Why do you think thoughts have increased?

If you find yourself thinking back to the co-emergence model, you are on the right track. When we sweep attention through the whole body, we feel many sensations in quick succession, and because of this, there will be many more co-emerging thoughts. This is an expected effect of this practice; you are not less skillful! By feeling all these sensations and the co-emerging thoughts with equanimity without reacting to them in any way, you are using a powerful desensitization method, and sensations and thoughts lose their power over you. Your internal experience and actions are no longer influenced by them. For example, memories of your past become just that—memories—and they lose their ability to drive and influence your behavior.

## How Attachment Results in Dissatisfaction

At this point of the advanced body scanning practices, you might notice that in some of your practice sessions there may be a few seconds or minutes when sensations feel very pleasant, even blissful. These can consciously or subconsciously remind us of past situations when we have felt similar pleasant sensations, such as what may occur during "flow states" like exercise, sexual activity, or creative endeavors.

With sweeping *en masse*, we can sometimes be surprised by a sense of having lost the solidity of the body or our sense of self. This can be very pleasant. But it is important to prevent attachment to this sense of "freedom from the body," just as it is important not to fear it. Sometimes people want to stay in this state as long as possible because it is very peaceful, but clinging to it only leads to craving it when it is absent.

As pleasant as these moments can be, it's essential not to cling to the sensations or the meaning we might assign to them. Although they may feel transformative and can offer a valuable perspective on life, attachment to any experience, blissful or otherwise, can impede your progress in developing equanimity. Just observe this momentary experience with equanimity and you will get the benefits without the disappointment when it doesn't return during your next meditation.

Experiences such as these can offer insight into how limited our day-to-day view of ourselves can be. Bringing this broader perspective to both how we relate to our ideas about ourselves, as well as to our interactions with others, can be very valuable, as we explain below.

# Interpersonal Mindfulness

You may have noticed how uncomfortable emotions and the associated unpleasant sensations can lead to avoiding not just specific situations or activities, as we addressed in stage 2, but also to avoiding conversations or interactions. This interpersonal avoidance—whether stemming from fear of criticism, rejection, conflict, or other concerns—might offer temporary relief, but it also breeds isolation, which is fertile ground for anxiety or depression to grow.

Consider your own experiences. Perhaps you've avoided a family gathering for fear of being judged, or dodged a conversation with a friend who seems to dismiss your views or feelings. Sometimes we avoid interactions with others to prevent our own anger. While such avoidance might feel like the safe route to take in the moment, it can deepen feelings of resentment, or a sense of being unwanted or unliked, thus perpetuating core beliefs that accompany anxiety and depression.

Remember that we are talking about addressing unhelpful patterns of avoidance here, such as avoiding meeting new people, or avoiding speaking to a neighbor about an issue with the recycling. There are other kinds of situations that are skillful to avoid, such as when someone is engaging in behavior that could endanger you.

This week, you're going to confront this pattern directly. Stage 3 of MiCBT will guide you to respond, not react, to others' emotional states. This is a powerful step. Understanding and acknowledging others' feelings, including their reactivity, without allowing it to influence your own emotional equilibrium, can transform your experience of these interactions.

## What Is Avoided in Interpersonal Interactions?

Have you ever avoided situations or interactions with people that you anticipate will feel uncomfortable? Especially when previous interactions were unpleasant, it's tempting to avoid certain people, which can lead to strained or absent communication. Future interactions can then feel even more awkward or otherwise challenging!

What exactly are we avoiding when we avoid interpersonal interactions? If we look within during these uncomfortable situations, we experience one thing in common in all of them: we feel unpleasant sensations in the body. When you realize that your reaction, such as avoiding interacting with that person, stems from your avoidance of unpleasant body sensations, it becomes easier to take responsibility for how you feel. And real empowerment comes from accepting responsibility for what you feel, including responsibility for any unpleasant sensations.

If you attribute your discomfort to external triggers—say, to someone else's judgment or attitude—you disempower yourself, because it implies that your discomfort can only end when that person stops judging you or changes their behavior. You depend on the other to feel better. On the other hand, if you can take experiential ownership, you will understand that no one else but you has the power to create the unpleasant sensations you feel in your body during these interactions. Therefore, only you can free yourself from them—and you *do* have this capability.

Of course, this applies to everyone else as well. Others, too, are producing their own body sensations and are responsible for them, even if you were an involuntary trigger for their discomfort. They may not have had opportunities yet to learn about the relationship between their thoughts, beliefs, and bodily sensations, and may be caught up in reactivity to sensations without even realizing it.

By taking responsibility for your experience, you can face previously challenging interpersonal situations with equanimity and wisdom, while reducing the tendency to avoid them. These are exactly the skills you will learn this week—understanding others' reactivity, and setting emotional boundaries during interpersonal interactions.

## Applying Your Skills: Experiential Ownership

*Experiential ownership* is a method that applies your mindfulness skills, especially equanimity, to sensations that co-emerge in interpersonally difficult situations. For instance, you might need to remind your children that it is bedtime, or express a difficult "no" to a loved one. Or you might need to spend time with someone around whom you feel awkward or otherwise uncomfortable. Other valuable opportunities to develop our mindfulness skills using experiential ownership include being around others who are in conflict, such as difficult workplace meetings where we experience unpleasant sensations, even though we are not directly involved. Note that experiential ownership is not about creating new conflicts in order to have opportunities to practice. Rather, we apply the four steps of experiential ownership to *existing* or *inevitable* tensions.

See the text box on the following page for step-by-step instructions to implement experiential ownership.

# Experiential Ownership

Experiential ownership can be practiced directly in daily life, or first using bipolar exposure, especially if you expect that the situation will be very challenging. This helps you start to desensitize to some extent before practicing it during an intense situation. When using experiential ownership in daily life, start directly with Step 1. If practicing using bipolar exposure beforehand, an ideal time is after practicing sweeping *en masse*.

## Setting Up Bipolar Exposure

Close your eyes, to help increase the vividness of your visualization and the intensity of co-emerging sensations.

Think of someone in your life that you have or expect to have challenging interactions with: someone who, when you visualize a difficult conversation with them, you know you will have unpleasant co-emerging sensations. Choose a fairly easy situation to work with to begin with, and when you feel more skilled and confident, progressively put yourself in more challenging ones.

Picture yourself in the location where you would typically have a difficult interaction with the person. Maybe it's at home, or at work... Where are you standing or sitting? Where is the other person? What is going on around the two of you? Are there any sounds or smells?

And now imagine you are experiencing the difficult interaction... It is getting more intense... Take some time to feel the co-emerging sensations arise...and now, start step 1 of experiential ownership. First, imagine the worst-case scenarios for five minutes; then, take a one-minute break to practice mindfulness of breath; and then visualize the best-case scenarios for five minutes.

## Step 1: Take Responsibility for Your Experience

- Scan through your body and locate the area of greatest intensity of sensations.

- Pay attention to the temperature, mass, motion, and density in this area, and apply full equanimity to these four building blocks of sensation within two seconds, regardless of whether they are pleasant, unpleasant, or neutral.

- Welcome these sensations, with a real willingness to feel them as they are, and NOT as part of a bargain to decrease them or make them more tolerable in some way.

- Take full responsibility for these sensations, as nobody can make you feel things in your body.

- Take "ownership" of your internal experience.

## Step 2: Recognize the Other Person's Experience

- Redirect your attention fully to the other person's experience.

- Notice their body language, the tone and pitch of their voice, without making any judgments.

- Try to guess what physical sensations they might be feeling in the moment (temperature, mass, motion, density).

- If they are being reactive, remind yourself that they are reacting to their co-emerging sensations, not the situation.

- Recognize that they may lack awareness of their habitual reactivity towards unpleasant, co-emerging body sensations, and may not be able to manage their inner experience with equanimity.

- Remind yourself that this person would probably not be reactive if they had had the benefit of training in equanimity.

## Step 3: Relinquish Responsibility for the Other's Experience

- Now disown responsibility for the other person's internal experience. The other person is responsible for the sensations that co-emerge with *their* thoughts in *their* bodies. They may be unaware that it is their thoughts and physical sensations that produce their discomfort, and yet this does not make you responsible for it.

- Don't react to their reactivity. You can accept the way the other person feels and reacts because you can see the co-emergence model "in action." That is, you can recognize how the meaning they assign to the situation leads them to feel intense sensations, which they then react to. Therefore, it does not make sense to take their reactivity personally.

## Step 4: Offer a Helpful Response

- Offer a helpful response: This might be a non-verbal acknowledgment or perhaps saying something that does not fuel further reactivity. If you can say something kind, that's even better!

Let's see what applying experiential ownership might look like during a disagreement with a friend. In step 1, you may notice a rapid heartbeat and a knot in your stomach. Instead of blaming your friend for how you feel, you accept that these sensations co-emerged with beliefs and thoughts in your own mind and feel them with equanimity, knowing that they will pass. Taking responsibility for them, in other words, taking "ownership," further empowers you to feel and accept these sensations, rather than avoid them.

Moving to step 2, you then focus on your friend, observing their body language, tone of voice, and choice of words. You might notice the redness in their cheeks or raised voice, reflecting their distress. You understand that they are feeling co-emerging sensations due to their thoughts and the meaning they assign to the situation, rather than directly because of you.

In step 3, you "disown" their experience, understanding that they are responsible for their co-emerging sensations, just as you are for yours. This does not mean you are indifferent to their feelings, but rather that you understand that you can't control their emotions any more than they can control yours.

Finally, in step 4, you might say "We don't have to talk about this now," or some other response that does not fuel reactivity. In week 8 you will learn the "seven statements of assertiveness" that you will use to ask for what you need, in those instances in which that is the preferred option—but for this week, simply offer a neutral response.

By taking responsibility for your experience, recognizing the experience of the other person, relinquishing responsibility for their experience (for example, not feeling guilty, ashamed, or angry), and offering a thoughtful response, you can be deeply aware of your and their emotional boundaries and maintain your equanimity during challenging interactions.

## This Week's Practice

During the practice of sweeping *en masse*, remember to bring an equal, curious, equanimous attention to both pleasant and unpleasant sensations. Even very pleasant experiences will pass—feel their pleasantness while they are present, but without attachment!

This week, put yourself in at least three situations with people which are safe, but you expect will still create some discomfort in either or both of you, and practice experiential ownership during these challenging interactions. Experiential ownership will serve as an important foundation for the seven statements of assertiveness that you'll be learning next week, so it is important that you practice it frequently, even in mildly uncomfortable interactions with people, to get to know the four steps very well. Refer back to these steps several times during the week to review them in detail.

When first practicing experiential ownership, choose situations that are less intense, so that you can apply equanimity to the co-emerging sensations more easily. As you become familiar with the steps and have some practice, you can start to use experiential ownership during more and more intense interpersonal situations.

After you've had a chance to practice experiential ownership in real life one or two times, come back to this workbook and write about the experience.

_____

_____

_____

_____

_____

_____

_____

_____

_____

---

## Week 7 Checklist

☐ Sweeping *en masse*: _____ / 14

    ☐ Audio Track 18: listen for the first two practices only

    ☐ Audio Track 19: listen with each practice

    ☐ Daily Record of Sweeping *en Masse* Practice

☐ Experiential ownership in challenging interactions: at least three times

## Daily Record of Sweeping en Masse Practice

| Day | Date | Morning Practice | Duration (Minutes) | Equanimity Rating Rate from 1 to 10 how much equanimity you had while feeling body sensations. 1 = minimal; 10 = full | Evening Practice | Duration (Minutes) | Equanimity Rating Rate from 1 to 10 how much equanimity you had while feeling body sensations. 1 = minimal; 10 = full |
|---|---|---|---|---|---|---|---|
| Day 1 | | yes / no | | | yes / no | | |
| Day 2 | | yes / no | | | yes / no | | |
| Day 3 | | yes / no | | | yes / no | | |
| Day 4 | | yes / no | | | yes / no | | |
| Day 5 | | yes / no | | | yes / no | | |
| Day 6 | | yes / no | | | yes / no | | |
| Day 7 | | yes / no | | | yes / no | | |

# Improving Communication in Relationships

Welcome to week 8, where we integrate advanced mindfulness skills with assertive communication. Together with the nonverbal skills you've been honing, we introduce "mindful assertiveness," using seven statements of assertiveness to help you express your views and needs safely, confidently, and respectfully. We also progress to "transversal scanning," during which you will learn to deepen your awareness of body sensations, further equipping you to confront and defuse deep-seated patterns of emotional reactivity.

## Review of Last Week's Practices

Looking back on your practice of sweeping *en masse* last week, were you able to move your attention through the whole body in a single flow of attention? It's OK if there were still some blank or vague spots that you needed to return to after sweeping, as that is also a valuable part of the process.

If you felt subtle, pleasant sensations throughout your body, were you able to remain equanimous? Perhaps you noticed more equanimity arising spontaneously during daily life as well, as the brain that we have when practicing meditation is the same brain we have during the rest of the day! As we've seen elsewhere in this program, benefits of skill training generalize into other areas of our life.

Did you notice having more intrusive thoughts during sweeping *en masse*? Were you able to remember that this is caused by feeling large areas of the body rapidly, which is accompanied by the co-emergence of many more thoughts? Could you remain equanimous and prevent judging yourself? Remember, this is always work in progress and gets better with practice.

If you feel a free flow of attention in some areas of the body, even just some of the time in your practice, you are ready to progress to transversal scanning. If not, continue to practice sweeping *en masse* for a few more days, this time in silence, with strong determination. The increased effort that this requires will help you notice more subtle sensations.

# Transversal Scanning

*Transversal scanning* extends feeling sensations to areas deep inside the body, so that "no stone remains unturned," so to speak. To achieve this, you'll be moving attention horizontally through the body, rather than vertically down the surface of the body.

Transversal scanning increases the likelihood of feeling very subtle sensations deep within the body, which may be linked to memories and emotions that you have not had the opportunity to desensitize to yet. Remaining aware and equanimous with all body sensations during transversal scanning allows even subconscious memories and associated habitual patterns of behavior (schemas) to be reexperienced with equanimity.

This creates a "prediction error mismatch." The brain is expecting the memory or belief to be experienced with distress, as it always has been, but it is now being experienced with non-reactivity and calmness instead. This results in the schema or memory being reconsolidated in memory *without* the same emotional charge (Ecker 2018). In the future, when the memory arises again, it is no longer associated with the same emotional charge or beliefs. By removing the reactivity associated with a distressing memory and reassociating the memory with equanimity, it becomes desensitized. We no longer live in the past!

## Practice Instructions

In transversal scanning, we start from the forehead, moving your attention horizontally *through* to the back of the head. Do your best to feel all the areas as you move attention toward the back. Continue to scan the rest of the head from front to back, part by part, with areas of attention about two to three inches in diameter.

When you have finished moving your attention from front to back, reverse the direction of attention, now scanning from the back of the head to the front. Once you have completed scanning the entire head from front to back and back to front, continue with the throat and neck, followed by each upper limb from shoulders to fingertips, feeling whatever sensations you can feel within the limb itself. The audio instructions will guide you to continue with the torso, and so on. When you reach the feet, return to the top of the head in the same way, and continue cycling through the body with equanimity for the entire thirty-minute practice. Remember that every sensation is impermanent and does not make up an "I," "me," or "mine."

Deep interoceptive desensitization is very effective, and change in our day-to-day life becomes clearly visible. We become more able to maintain equanimity, even during challenging interactions.

# Mindful Assertiveness

Assertiveness training has been a part of transdiagnostic mental health treatment approaches for decades. The goal of assertiveness training is to help you communicate your thoughts, feelings, and needs effectively and respectfully, in a way that acknowledges the rights and feelings of others while also advocating for your own rights and needs.

Introducing more assertiveness into how we communicate with others can feel especially difficult in the context of recent or current depression and anxiety. It has been known for decades that challenges with assertiveness are often associated with heightened social anxiety, diminished self-esteem, and increased depressive symptoms and avoidance behavior.

When we're anxious or depressed, we are especially prone to getting caught up in distorted beliefs such as, *If I say what I want, others will think I'm selfish*, or *It's my duty to please others, even at the cost of my own needs.* You may find yourself being overly cautious in interactions with others, fearing that expressing yourself may upset them, or they might reject you. Or you might be unrealistically rigid in your expectations of others, and feel justified in becoming angry when you perceive them as not meeting their commitments.

What do both ends of this spectrum have in common with each other? You may have noticed from stage 1 and stage 2 that the co-emergence model applies here as well! It is reactivity to co-emerging sensations that propels us to either not speak up or become angry. And if you recall, these sensations are the consequence of how we evaluate the situation when it has meaning or significance for "me"—the "I," "me," or "mine." When we're reacting to these sensations, we're much more likely to say something more softly and timidly, or more loudly and aggressively than intended. The other person will in turn react to our attitude—to *how* we said something—rather than paying attention to *what* we need them to hear. Instead, by integrating your experiential ownership skills with assertive communication based on the co-emergence model, you'll develop *mindful assertiveness*, which can be defined as the ability to communicate clearly and confidently while remaining equanimous with one's internal state.

## Finding a Mutually Convenient Time to Talk

Before diving into a potentially challenging conversation, you need to pick the right moment for it. Imagine your friend engrossed in their favorite book. Interrupting them could lead them to feel irritated, making them less receptive to your concerns. Valuing their time by checking in with them to find a mutually convenient time to talk sets a respectful atmosphere. Once you have found a good time to talk, you are almost ready to go!

## The Importance of Experiential Ownership

Just as the walls of a house need a solid foundation to stay upright, experiential ownership provides stable, reliable ground for you to stand on when expressing your views and needs. Last week you practiced bringing equanimity to intense sensations during uncomfortable interpersonal situations while taking full responsibility for your own experience, and recognizing the other person's reactivity with empathy, without taking responsibility for it.

If there were no opportunities to practice experiential ownership last week, hold off on starting mindful assertiveness for a few days. Becoming familiar with the experiential ownership process is crucial for assertiveness to be expressed mindfully.

Remember to implement experiential ownership each time you use the seven statements of assertiveness. If you find that you're too agitated and not able to bring equanimity to areas of intense body sensations, then we suggest that you delay your conversation. It would not be productive to ask for what you want or express your views in an emotionally reactive manner, as it would only serve to reinforce habits of reactivity.

## Applying Your Skills: Seven Statements of Assertiveness

The *seven statements of assertiveness* listed below provide a clear and easy-to-use framework to express your views and needs effectively and respectfully. Let's look at each of them with an example of how they can be applied:

1. **State the facts:** Begin by clearly stating the facts, stripped of exaggeration, blame, or emotional coloring. Let's use a common household scenario as an example. Instead of accusing your roommate, "You never take out the trash," you could state the facts: "Taking out the trash is on your list of shared household chores, and it hasn't been taken out in two weeks." By steering clear of absolute terms like "never" or "always," you are more likely to present the situation as it is, without misrepresentation. This keeps the line of communication open and lessens the chance of the other person feeling judged.

2. **State how you feel:** The next step involves expressing your emotions clearly and honestly. It is crucial to differentiate between projecting your emotions onto the other person and owning your feelings. For example, instead of saying "You make me angry when you don't keep your commitments," express your feelings using "I" statements, such as "Every time this happens, I feel frustrated." This approach invites empathy rather than reactivity, such as defensiveness.

3. **State how or what you think:** Now, connect your feelings to the thoughts behind them. Sharing what you think gives a more accurate context to your emotions. Instead of blaming

the other person by saying, "Because I didn't complain in the past, now you're taking me for granted," you could express your thought process as: "I feel frustrated because it seems to me that I'm not important enough to you for you to remember our agreement." This shows the other person that you are taking responsibility for what you feel, as you link your disappointment to your own evaluation rather than the actions of the other person. Not blaming the other person for what you feel will help them listen to the content of your message. Your mantra this week is: *My message must be louder than me*, and not the other way around, or no one will hear it.

4.  **State your possible error in judgment:** This step involves humility and self-awareness. It is about recognizing that your perspective might be flawed due to your own biases and past experiences. In this example, instead of rigidly holding onto your view, you could say, "I could be misinterpreting why you don't take the trash out." This openness to the possibility of being wrong in your interpretation of the situation can reduce misunderstandings and invite constructive feedback.

5.  **State what you want:** Expressing your needs and desires is crucial. Instead of saying, "It's not fair that I have to put up with bad smells and flies when you don't stick to what we agree," state what you need: "I can't do both our chores, and I really need you to commit to doing yours. Can you ensure that you'll take the trash out regularly?" By kindly and equanimously putting forth what you want, you offer a clear pathway towards a solution, shifting the conversation from complaints to constructive action.

6.  **Thank the person if cooperation occurs:** Positive reinforcement in the form of appreciation can go a long way in nurturing healthy relationships. If the other person has agreed to your request, provide a rewarding response by thanking them and expressing your genuine gratitude. Then you are done—there is no need to move on to Step 7. But things won't always go your way, despite your kindest approach! They may not agree to your request, perhaps saying "Taking out the trash is not a big issue. I mean, really…is that big of a deal?" You can still thank them for taking the time to listen to you, as this will help them be more likely to listen to your concerns in the future. For example, you can say "Thanks for making time to talk about this" and then move to Step 7.

7.  **Negotiate (discuss a win-win solution):** If disagreements remain, work towards a mutually beneficial solution, or at least a mutually least unfavorable one. You could propose the following: "I understand it can be difficult to remember tasks that seem trivial to you, but having an overflowing garbage is not hygienic and can attract rats, and I don't have time to do all the

chores by myself. Let's find a compromise that respects both our needs. Perhaps we could swap tasks? I could be in charge of the trash and you vacuuming?" Remember, not all issues can be resolved perfectly, but the goal is to find a solution that respects everyone's needs.

## Applying the Seven Statements of Assertiveness

Let's picture a scenario where a work colleague, who is going through a difficult separation, has been repeatedly speaking to you and others in a rude and demeaning way for the past three months. The whole team has been tolerant and patient, but eventually, you decide to speak privately with your colleague.

**Find a mutually convenient time to talk:** Hey, I need to have a quick chat with you about something for a few minutes—is now a good time? Great, thanks.

1.  **State the facts:** I noticed that over the past three months you've been speaking with me in a way that I find hurtful. We used to be friendly with each other, and this has clearly changed.

2.  **State how you feel:** Since then, I've been feeling anxious and sometimes frustrated around you...

3.  **State how or what you think:** ...because I think that you might react negatively at any time, and maybe our friendship is over.

4.  **State your possible error in judgment:** I might be wrong about this, and if so, I apologize, but...

5.  **State what you want:** I want for us to go back to being more at ease with each other. Perhaps you could trust me enough to share what's really on your mind when you get frustrated, rather than having me walk on eggshells. Can we make that happen?

6.  **Thank them for their cooperation:** Thanks for understanding. I really appreciate it, and I'm happy to listen and talk about anything that might be helpful.

Take a moment to write down a scenario from your own life where using mindful assertiveness would be beneficial. Then, using the framework of the seven assertive statements above, write out what you would say. Keep statements brief.

Describe the scenario briefly: _____

_____

Find a mutually convenient time to talk: _____

_____

1. State the facts: _____

_____

_____

2. State how you feel: _____

_____

_____

3. State how or what you think: _____

_____

_____

4. State your possible error in judgment: _____

_____

_____

5. State what you want: _____

_____

_____

_____

**6. Thank the other for their cooperation:** _____

_____

_____

**7. Negotiate (discuss a win-win solution, if required):** _____

_____

_____

## This Week's Practice

When practicing transversal scanning twice daily this week, you may find that the speed of scanning slows down significantly. This is to be expected, as you are returning to part-by-part scanning. At the beginning of the week, you may find that it takes the whole practice session to scan from the top of the head to the toes. This is not a problem. Simply start your next practice at the feet and move up to the head part-by-part.

Remember to always accompany the seven statements of assertiveness with experiential ownership, as this will preserve your equanimity as well as good emotional boundaries. And just like with experiential ownership last week, the seven statements of assertiveness can be practiced using bipolar exposure prior to having the actual conversation in real life.

---

### Week 8 Checklist

☐ Transversal scanning: _____/14

    ☐ Audio Track 20: listen for the first two practices only

    ☐ Audio Track 21: listen with each practice

    ☐ Daily Record of Transversal Scanning Practice

☐ Implement the seven statements of assertiveness with equanimity at least twice this week

## Daily Record of Transversal Scanning Practice

| Day | Date | Morning Practice | Duration (Minutes) | Equanimity Rating Rate from 1 to 10 how much equanimity you had while feeling body sensations. 1 = minimal; 10 = full | Evening Practice | Duration (Minutes) | Equanimity Rating Rate from 1 to 10 how much equanimity you had while feeling body sensations. 1 = minimal; 10 = full |
|---|---|---|---|---|---|---|---|
| Day 1 | | yes / no | | | yes / no | | |
| Day 2 | | yes / no | | | yes / no | | |
| Day 3 | | yes / no | | | yes / no | | |
| Day 4 | | yes / no | | | yes / no | | |
| Day 5 | | yes / no | | | yes / no | | |
| Day 6 | | yes / no | | | yes / no | | |
| Day 7 | | yes / no | | | yes / no | | |

# Developing Compassion

As we begin week 9, we progress to stage 4 of MiCBT, where we focus on cultivating compassion and decreasing relapse into depression and anxiety. As anxiety and depression can contribute to feeling disconnected from yourself or others, you'll learn to develop the power of loving-kindness meditation and ethical awareness to restore your sense of connection and community. Additionally, you'll be introduced to the final advanced scanning technique, "sweeping in depth," to further develop equanimity.

## Review of Last Week's Practices

Were you able to scan your body transversally, maintaining equanimity even with blank spots? In parallel with this, you might also have noticed that you are less reactive when things don't go the way you would prefer during daily life. How about communicating with mindful assertiveness? Regardless of the outcome, the process of maintaining equanimity with co-emerging body sensations while sharing your view or asking for what you want is a powerful way to train equanimity. Over time, as you become more familiar with the seven statements, you may find yourself spontaneously incorporating them into your day-to-day conversations, using your own style.

You are ready to move to the next step when you can feel at least forty percent of the interior of the body. If this is not yet possible, practice transversal scanning for several more days, this time without audio instructions, to get more benefit from the next practice, sweeping in depth. If you struggle with many thoughts during practice, start with ten minutes of mindfulness of breath and resume transversal scanning for the remaining twenty minutes.

## Sweeping in Depth

This fifth and final advanced body scanning practice is called *sweeping in depth*, which combines transversal scanning and sweeping *en masse*. By combining feeling sensations throughout the body, including inside, with a sweeping vertical movement of attention, you will develop the ability to feel sensations throughout the body very quickly, eventually in the space of a single breath. As you train this skill during meditation, you will increasingly notice very early signs of reactivity in daily life, allowing you to prevent your reactions before they grow and lead you to manifest them behaviorally. Feeling sensations deeply and rapidly while remaining equanimous can also improve your understanding of your deepest emotions and their origins.

## Practice Instructions

Begin by focusing your attention at the top of your head and practice sweeping *en masse*, while also moving your attention through the interior of the body to the toes, feeling as many sensations as possible both at the surface of the body and within it. After reaching the toes, reverse direction and sweep upward to the top of the head in a single flow of attention, again feeling as much as possible on your way.

If you encounter areas where sensations are absent or faint, note the location, but continue sweeping. After two or three complete sweeps, return to these blank or unclear spots and survey them, part by part, before returning to sweeping. If feeling internal sensations using sweeping is challenging through most of the body, combine this technique with transversal scanning: one body cycle of transversal scanning, followed by two or three cycles of sweeping in depth. Continue this combination throughout your thirty-minute practice.

# Purpose of Compassion Training

Compassion is the urge, the wish to take action to relieve suffering, whether someone else's or your own. Compassion extends beyond empathy and intellectual understanding; it is a felt experience in the body. Compassion propels us towards kind intention and action. It can take the form of something we do or say, or the thoughts or intentions we have. Compassion for yourself and others is an ideal solution for preventing relapse into depression, because you can't be genuinely kind to yourself and others while at the same time criticizing, blaming, or hating yourself or others. Negative rumination and compassion can't live together!

It is normal to feel sensations of discomfort ourselves when we witness another's suffering. "Mirror neurons" in the brain imitate the other person's experience and cause us to feel what we believe the other is feeling. Our brain is naturally wired to make us care about each other.

However, caring a lot about people who suffer, without maintaining a degree of equanimity, can result in emotional exhaustion and sometimes burnout. To be experienced productively, compassion needs to be accompanied by both equanimity and mindful discernment. Equanimity allows us to be receptive to suffering, experiencing the unpleasant sensations it can incite within the body without aversion or distress. Mindful discernment guides us to act skillfully to alleviate suffering. Moreover, equanimity prevents attachment to the outcome of our compassionate actions, thereby lessening disappointment when we don't get the results we hoped for.

Compassion for yourself is just as important as compassion for others. Research has shown that improvement in self-compassion after eight weeks of mindfulness training is associated with reductions in anxiety and depressed mood (ter Avest et al. 2021). Anxiety and low mood can worsen by identifying with setbacks and perceived failures; by training to be more compassionate, you cultivate self-acceptance in a way that lessens the self-critical thoughts so common in depression. This compassionate approach allows you to see your struggles as part of the universal human experience, fostering a sense of connection, and reducing feelings of isolation.

## Loving-Kindness Practice

To develop compassion, teachers of mindfulness and wisdom have taught loving-kindness meditation for the past twenty-six centuries. In MiCBT, loving-kindness is also an important means of developing compassion. We use the subtle sensations that we feel in the body following the practice of sweeping in depth as the starting point for "embodying" our compassion practice. We begin by *feeling* body sensations co-emerging with kind wishes for our well-being, and then pair this felt experience of kindness in the body with other compassionate thoughts. Grounding compassion practice in the body helps us remember to remain compassionate during daily life.

Loving-kindness meditation is practiced for about ten minutes after the thirty-minute body scanning practice twice daily. To practice it, follow the audio instructions that guide you through these three steps:

1. **Self-compassion:** Begin with focusing your attention at the center of your chest, feeling sensations in this "heart" area. If feeling sensations in this area is difficult, focus on other parts of the body where pleasant sensations might be easier to feel, such as the palms of the hands. With each inhalation, feel the pleasant sensations, and with each exhalation, feel these sensations spreading throughout your entire body. If feeling them is difficult at this early stage of practice, you can imagine them until you become more able to feel them. Simultaneously, formulate kind wishes for your well-being, grounding these intentions in your bodily experience. As per the audio guide, these include affirmations such as "May I be peaceful," "May I be kind to myself," and "May I feel joy and contentment."

2. **Compassion for loved ones:** Continue to feel any pleasant, warm sensations in the center of the chest area, or other part of the body, with each inhalation. With each exhalation, let these sensations infused with your compassionate intentions radiate out towards those you care for.

Along with this, formulate compassionate wishes for them. As per the audio guide, these include "May you be at ease," "May you be free from reactivity," and "May you be happy."

3. **Compassion for all beings:** Maintain your attention on the sensations in the chest area as you inhale. Upon exhaling, let these sensations spread outward in all directions to all beings. This can include animals and plants as well. Develop benevolent thoughts for all beings, recognizing that everyone is subject to suffering. As per the audio guide, these affirmations include "May all beings be free from harm," "May all beings be peaceful," and "May all beings be free from suffering."

# Working with Habitual Negative Beliefs

As you practice loving-kindness meditation, you may encounter habitual negative beliefs about yourself, such as *I don't deserve to be happy* or *I can't imagine saying this to myself.* If you feel some resistance to extending well-wishes to yourself, bring equanimity to even this, being careful to not identify with these types of thoughts and their co-emerging sensations.

Remember when you first started body scanning, and there were areas of the body where it was hard to feel any sensations? Chances are that now you do feel subtle or even prominent sensations in those areas! Similarly, loving-kindness practice can initially be challenging, especially when depressive or anxiety symptoms have been present for some time, or your sense of self-worth is still low. However, much like the body scanning, if you persist with the intention to eventually feel and accept this kindness, and remain equanimous when you don't, you will find yourself able to start to feel genuine compassion toward yourself. We can even feel compassionate towards ourselves when habitual negative beliefs about ourselves or others arise. By reprocessing these beliefs within this compassionate and caring awareness, we change our relationship with our self-beliefs.

During loving-kindness practice, feelings of sadness, regret, anger, or resentment may surface. Navigating forgiveness can feel like a complex task. As we explored in chapter 3, we can recognize these self-criticisms as part of a larger pattern of human suffering, rather than personal shortcomings.

Finally, loving-kindness practice is a powerful tool for developing disidentification with the self. There's no distinct, separate self to cherish or resent; instead, the practice of mindfulness meditation uncovers the impermanent nature of our identity. Sensations are not of a "self," but merely of a body. Over time, this becomes clearer. As these insights mature, you may notice that deep-seated negative beliefs such as *I'm unworthy* or *I'm doomed to fail* start to lose their grip. This not only reduces the severity of depressive or anxious symptoms but also fosters a greater sense of compassion and understanding towards yourself and others.

## Modifications to Loving-Kindness Practice

It can sometimes feel challenging to extend a feeling of well-wishing to ourselves or to specific individuals. This might be particularly true if you've grown up in an environment lacking warmth and affection, or if there has been a history of abuse. In such instances, you might feel reluctant to extend compassion, perhaps feeling unworthy or anxious about self-compassion, or angry about past injustices. Using some of the approaches below, you can adapt the loving-kindness practice to your unique needs:

1. **Gradual inclusion of self-compassion:** Rather than starting with loving-kindness for yourself, start by recalling individuals who have been kind to you. Begin by thinking about, and then feeling, a sense of gratitude for their contributions to your well-being, or other positive actions they've taken. Once you can feel pleasant sensations associated with this sense of gratitude, gradually extend the feeling of gratitude towards your own efforts to help yourself, even ones that may seem small. In this way, step by step, you gradually move from gratitude towards others, to gratitude towards self, and to a more unconditional acceptance of yourself and others.

2. **Working with difficult relationships:** Perhaps there is someone in your life with whom you've had a challenging relationship, or whose views you disagree with strongly. If including them in your practice feels too difficult, it is okay to exclude them initially. If you do choose to include them at some point, you could begin by cultivating the wish for them to gain insight into their actions and develop their own kindness and compassion.

## Applying Your Skills: Ethical Conduct as Compassion

Imagine this—you're working hard, practicing loving-kindness twice daily, and making real progress, cultivating compassion for yourself and others. But one day, you find yourself in a heated argument with a family member. They're angry and their words sting. You're feeling attacked and your mind is racing with thoughts like *Why do they always blame me?* or *Nobody ever listens to my side of the story!* These thoughts are like adding fuel to a fire—their heat is turning into unpleasant body sensations.

What if you could remember your loving-kindness practice right then and there during the argument, tapping into that space of compassion, and choose a response that doesn't harm you or your family member? Compassionate action for both yourself and others can take the form of ethical conduct motivated by kindness and nonviolence.

This week, we'll be practicing applying compassion "in the heat of the moment" by preventing five types of harmful actions: using harmful speech, taking what is not yours or hasn't been given to you, being physically harmful, engaging in sexual misconduct, and consuming intoxicants.

1. **Using helpful speech:** Aim to foster truthful, timely, and respectful communication. Maintain awareness of your speech throughout the day, and consider five guidelines before you speak: Is it true? Is it kind? Is it necessary? Is it timely? Is it useful? Also, remember to avoid divisive, backbiting, or misleading speech. Speaking truthfully with equanimity can be empowering for all.

2. **Taking what is freely given:** Taking what is not given mostly occurs because of craving or unawareness of the consequence to others. Being careful to only take what is freely given prevents the reinforcement of craving. This doesn't just refer to physical things. For example, we can habitually take time or attention from others, sometimes without even intending to.

3. **Refraining from taking life:** This third domain invites us to not take lives voluntarily. For example, consider not killing insects in bathtubs, and being mindful while wiping down a picnic table to avoid killing ants. These are small opportunities to practice non-harming. Practicing kindness reinforces mindfulness, and vice versa.

4. **Engaging in appropriate sexual actions:** Refraining from inappropriate sexual actions isn't limited to not affairs or overt acts of sexual violence. We can bring attention to subtle manifestations of craving, like flirting with someone when knowing that it could be hurtful to your committed partner. This behavior may provide temporary pleasant sensations, but it is also inconsistent with wishing your partner well during loving-kindness practice, and perpetuates craving.

5. **Refraining from intoxicants:** Avoiding substances that reduce your prefrontal cortex's self-control functions, like alcohol and cannabis, is helpful, as these substances compromise your ability to prevent harmful verbal or physical actions. When intoxicated, practicing compassion through the first four domains listed above becomes significantly more challenging, if at all possible.

It is important to understand that acting compassionately to prevent harm is not about rigidly adhering to a set of imposed rules out of fear or guilt, nor because our therapist suggested it, nor is it about "being a better person" in an effort to enhance our self-image. Choosing helpful speech, for example, isn't about striving to appear virtuous, or something you're expected to do even in the face of another person's aggressive or otherwise unhelpful speech. Instead, it is guided by a genuine intention to prevent causing harm to others and to yourself—as speech that is motivated by craving and aversion is mostly harmful.

In MiCBT, ethical action is about compassion-driven choices that aim to reduce suffering, and create an atmosphere of safety, trust, and mutual respect. This aspiration for compassionate action creates a sense of connection to others and your environment. Relapse into depression is less likely in the context of this sense of "wholesome connectedness."

## This Week's Practice

With consistent practice of sweeping in depth, the skill of being able to feel subtle sensations throughout the body will generalize into daily life, allowing you to feel with equanimity whatever is arising during even busy, intense moments of the day.

Training compassion during loving-kindness meditation and during the day in the form of ethical behavior in five specific domains will also generalize to other parts of your day. By paying very careful attention to your intentions and actions, you'll progressively be able to notice when subtle signs of aversion and craving are driving your behavior, and to make more skillful choices.

---

## Week 9 Checklist

☐ Sweeping in depth and loving-kindness practice: _____ /14

    ☐ Audio Track 20: for the first two practices only

    ☐ Audio Track 21: listen with each practice

    ☐ Daily Record of Sweeping in Depth and Loving-Kindness Practice

☐ Implement ethical awareness practices

    ☐ Daily Record of Ethical Awareness Practices

## Daily Record of Sweeping in Depth and Loving-Kindness Practice

| Day | Date | Morning Practice | Duration (Minutes) | Equanimity Rating<br>Rate from 1 to 10 how much equanimity you had while feeling body sensations.<br>1 = minimal; 10 = full | Evening Practice | Duration (Minutes) | Equanimity Rating<br>Rate from 1 to 10 how much equanimity you had while feeling body sensations.<br>1 = minimal; 10 = full |
|---|---|---|---|---|---|---|---|
| Day 1 | | yes / no | | | yes / no | | |
| Day 2 | | yes / no | | | yes / no | | |
| Day 3 | | yes / no | | | yes / no | | |
| Day 4 | | yes / no | | | yes / no | | |
| Day 5 | | yes / no | | | yes / no | | |
| Day 6 | | yes / no | | | yes / no | | |
| Day 7 | | yes / no | | | yes / no | | |

## Daily Record of Ethical Awareness Practices

| | Situation (Place, context, time) | Reaction or Response? (Were you able to prevent reactive behavior?) | Compassionate Action (Helpful speech, not stealing, not killing, appropriate sexual action, refraining from intoxicants) | How long did you apply effort for? | How do you feel now about your reaction or response during the experience? |
|---|---|---|---|---|---|
| Day 1 | | | | | |
| Day 2 | | | | | |
| Day 3 | | | | | |
| Day 4 | | | | | |
| Day 5 | | | | | |
| Day 6 | | | | | |
| Day 7 | | | | | |

# Cultivating Resilience and Well-Being

Congratulations! You've made it to your tenth and last week of the MiCBT program. Continuing your journey of self-discovery and wisdom, this chapter introduces ten priceless human qualities to further uproot the causes of depression and anxiety. You will also be introduced to the once daily "maintenance practice," which helps to maintain attention regulation, emotion regulation, and compassion skills, which in turn promote resilience and well-being. It is now time to move beyond therapy toward personal growth, becoming the architect of your future.

## Review of Last Week's Practices

How was your practice of sweeping in depth? Could you feel a free flow of soft tingling sensations in most of the body's interior? This can take some time to achieve and shouldn't be rushed. You can now take all the time you need to refine your skills.

And how was your practice of loving-kindness meditation and ethical living? Can you now feel a sense of being more connected within yourself and with others? This sense of connectedness is probably one of the greatest protective factors against relapse into depression and anxiety, so it is worth considering maintaining these practices.

## Review of Overall Progress

It is now time to reflect on your journey. One way of measuring general progress is to look at your experience of equanimity across various life contexts. If you are less reactive in most situations, you have definitely moved forward. There will be inevitable moments where you'll feel emotionally reactive, such as the justifiable fear for a gravely ill family member or the death of a beloved pet. However, in such situations, if you clearly notice that the length of reactivity is getting shorter, you are continuing to make progress.

## Measuring Equanimity

To gauge improvement in equanimity, revisit the Equanimity Scale-16, which you first completed in chapter 3. You can access and complete it again using the downloadable version (http://www.newharbinger.com/52571) and compare your current responses with your initial ones. We also recommend that you re-rate your *initial* scoring to see if you had filled it in accurately the first time. You may discover that your initial scores had been overly optimistic. Our research shows that as people develop more insight into their behavior and degree of equanimity, they become more realistic about their prior level of equanimity (Shires et al. 2023). This shift not only indicates growth in equanimity but is also a great sign of increased self-awareness.

## Overview of Skills Gained

During the MiCBT program, you developed skills across several domains of your life and learned to prevent the reinforcement of mechanisms underlying depression and anxiety.

You started with stage 1, focusing your attention internally to develop equanimity with thoughts and sensations. You learned to be less reactive and more aware and accepting of your internal experiences. This alone is likely to have made a positive difference in your life.

With stage 2, you learned to externalize these self-regulation skills to reduce avoidant behavior. In doing so, your equanimity and sense of confidence improved. Like many people, you may also have been surprised at how quickly your avoidance, however well established, can decrease.

You then began stage 3 and extended these skills into your interactions with others. You began to be more confident around people with whom there may have been some tension, and gained a better understanding and acceptance of their emotional reactivity, as well as the suffering it involves. This informed you about the nature of conflict between people, with the recognition that we react to our own internal experience, while assuming that the other person has caused our dissatisfaction. This stage is usually very beneficial for relationships.

Finally, in stage 4, you further extended your skills to become mindful of your own and others' goodness. By developing compassionate intentions and a kind attention to preventing harm to yourself and others, you may now be feeling more connected with the world. You may also have a sense of how "we are all in the same boat," so to speak, and how human beings can disengage from unnecessary suffering, influencing each other for the greater good.

It is common for people who develop these skills to feel gratitude. If you also feel grateful, it may be toward the person who recommended this program, or the supportive family members who made it possible for you to make time to practice every day. We, too, are grateful to our own teachers. Having gratitude for the skills you've gained is also a sign of progress, because you are mindful of others' helpful influences in your success, which in turn helps you feel connected to them. This sense of connectedness protects you from emotional distress. You can now better understand how we are at higher risk for depression and anxiety when we feel disconnected from others and from our own experiences, and how we can prevent this when we feel compassionate and connected.

## Review of Initial Targeted Problems and Success Indicators

Another way of measuring progress is to look back at your initial targeted problems and success indicators in chapter 1. In the table below, you can fill in the columns and rate from 1 to 10 to what extent you have been able to accomplish your success indicators. If all have been achieved to some degree, it's time to celebrate! If some continue to need work, acknowledge this, commit to working on them, and celebrate what you have already accomplished! After all, life will keep bringing more challenges, and the skills you have learned can be invaluable companions for years to come.

| Targeted Problems | Success Indicators | Improvement |
|---|---|---|
| 1. | A. | |
| | B. | |
| | C. | |
| 2. | A. | |
| | B. | |
| | C. | |

| Targeted Problems | Success Indicators | Improvement |
|---|---|---|
| 3. | A. | |
| | B. | |
| | C. | |
| 4. | A. | |
| | B. | |
| | C. | |
| 5. | A. | |
| | B. | |
| | C. | |

## Cultivating Resilience and Well-Being

Maintaining your skills is central to preventing relapse into depression and anxiety. It is also a very wholesome way of cultivating resilience and personal growth. To this end, we invite you to continue a daily maintenance practice of the skills you have learned.

## Maintenance Practice

To preserve the three main meditative skills which have benefited you so far, *maintenance practice* combines mindfulness of breath, body scanning, and loving-kindness into a once daily forty-five minute practice. The first ten minutes are dedicated to mindfulness of breath, the following twenty-five minutes are for body scanning, and the last ten minutes conclude the session with loving-kindness.

As you are now trained in these three methods, the audio guidance mostly serves as a timer and only cues you briefly at the start of each method, leaving most of the session for silent practice. This allows you to go deeper into your meditation without being distracted by audio instructions.

For many, morning practice is optimal due to increased energy and focus, making learning easier. Practicing forty-five minutes after dinner can be particularly challenging, leading to drowsiness and distractibility. Morning practice primes our skills for the day, making them readily accessible. After dedicating time twice a day over the past ten weeks, perhaps sacrificing time with family or friends, moving to a morning practice can free up precious evenings.

Maintenance practice offers many opportunities to recognize similarities between patterns of sensations you experience during meditation and those that arise in the body as you go about your day. All the work you have done learning to consistently apply equanimity to these sensations during meditation to prevent habitual reactivity has been generalizing to daily life as well. In other words, since you have the same brain in both contexts, correcting its habits in one will correct it in the other.

## Relapse Prevention and the Brain

The ability to prevent relapse depends greatly on patterns of neural connectivity. For example, over the last ten weeks you've strengthened connections between brain cells in the salience network by training the ability to feel body sensations while being intentional and objective in your interpretation of them. The salience network allows you to be aware of body sensations, among other functions. Keeping these areas of the brain well connected reduces feelings of dissociation from your body when anxious.

You may have also noticed that nowadays when emotional reactivity *does* occur, it doesn't last as long as it used to. This is related to two additional changes that occur in the brain with mindfulness meditation. The first is an improvement in functioning of the central executive network, which, like the conductor of an orchestra, coordinates activity in different parts of the brain (Bauer et al. 2019) and decisions and actions in our daily life. As a result, it's able to regulate default mode network activity (as we discussed in chapter 3) more effectively, resulting in less "I," "me," and "mine" thinking and shortened periods of reactivity.

Secondly, the right amygdala, a small almond-shaped structure located deep inside the limbic area of your brain, decreases in size, and this change has been associated with stress reduction (Holzel et al. 2010).

One of the ways this occurs is that equanimity helps inhibit overactivity in the amygdala. Relapse into depression and anxiety is more likely to occur if the amygdala is overactive, so maintaining your level of equanimity matters a lot.

# Deepening Wisdom and Well-Being

We now turn to a set of ten protective and wisdom-enhancing factors—beneficial human qualities, rooted in compassion for yourself and others—that can serve as fertilizers for your personal growth. Like the other skills you have been practicing in this program, these are not confined to your meditation practice; they can be practiced anytime and anywhere.

These skills effectively counteract habitual views that can hinder your progress or even invite anxiety and depression. The more you practice them, the better. There is no limit to the amount of wisdom, kindness, and other helpful skills you can cultivate.

## Generosity

Generosity extends far beyond the act of giving material possessions or monetary assistance. It encompasses offering time, skills, and attention. By willingly sharing what we have, we let go of related attachments and fears. In fact, generosity enhances our sense of friendliness, compassion, and self-worth, fostering a feeling of interconnectedness. This is because it reduces our focus on self, and lets us experience the joy of enriching the lives of those around us.

It is common to hear parents, in particular, say that they want to train in mindfulness to change and prevent "passing on" their depression, anxiety, irritability, or other types of suffering to their children. In this case, their practice of mindfulness meditation itself is an act of generosity. By investing personal effort in cultivating mindfulness, we alleviate suffering not just within ourselves but also in the lives of others.

## Preventing Harm (or Cultivating Virtue)

As we discussed in week 9, the intention to prevent harm to oneself and others out of compassion is another maturing factor. It is a virtuous intention and the actions that follow are a universal means of cultivating self-esteem. Respecting ethical boundaries and preventing harm, from a sense of care for yourself and others, will lead to feeling more worthy—which is a great antidote for rumination and self-criticism!

You may recall that a useful way of knowing whether your intentions are wholesome or unwholesome at a given time is to feel into co-emerging sensations at this moment. Remember that unwholesome thoughts co-emerge with unpleasant body sensations, whereas wholesome thoughts do not. Being able to act in helpful ways despite feeling unpleasant sensations is a great virtue!

## Renunciation

Renouncing means "letting go." Developing generosity and virtue first requires us to say "no," or "renounce" habits of being self-centered or acting in harmful ways. As such, renunciation is central to developing virtue and generosity, as well as other wholesome human qualities.

During mindfulness meditation, you practice renunciation every time you abandon a thought that enters your mind, you refuse to react when a very pleasant or unpleasant sensation occurs in your body, and you reject the idea that your sense of self is permanent. This is the deepest experiential aspect of renunciation.

In daily life, renunciation occurs every time we refuse to fall back into unhelpful old habits, such as ruminating, or using intoxicants. Renouncing old habits also means reducing both attachment to pleasure and craving for it when it is absent. In turn, this reduces the probability of being dissatisfied with our lives and relapsing into depression and anxiety. As you have probably guessed, renunciation is an essential aspect of self-control and an important element of equanimity.

## Insight (or Wisdom)

Wisdom can be understood as insight into the reality of a present moment, including its causes and future consequences. Wisdom therefore allows us to perceive in any given moment the most beneficial decision for all parties involved, in the short and long term. It is the ability to understand cause and effect and act in a way that prevents extremes and minimizes suffering.

Insight is not born from idealism. It is the result of continual effort to remain aware of the three universal causes of suffering that we discussed in chapter 2: craving, aversion, and the unawareness of impermanence, including that of our sense of self.

In the context of MiCBT, developing experiential wisdom is the greatest achievement. As wisdom develops, it becomes easier to avoid extremes and perceive a "middle way." For example, bringing wisdom to a conversation with someone who argues against your view will not stop you from being assertive (as you learned in stage 3) when it is skillful to do so, but you are also less likely to insist on sharing your perspective when it is not beneficial to do so. With wisdom, you know that "being right" doesn't necessarily make you happy.

## Effort

Without effort, not much happens. However, we can expend effort in unproductive or even destructive ways. To contribute to personal growth, your effort must be productive and genuinely beneficial. For example, the effort to maintain your daily meditation practice even when you are tired or unmotivated is genuinely beneficial. The effort to remain attentive and prevent drowsiness during meditation is also a wholesome effort, as it makes your meditation practice productive. The effort to be mindful of your thoughts, sensations, and intentions, and to remain ethical in daily life is equally beneficial.

## Patience

According to Ajahn Jayasaro (2010), "patience is an ability to peacefully co-exist with the unpleasant." For example, patience is needed to complete your entire meditation practice every day, and not stop it before the end if your experience becomes unpleasant. Patience aligns beautifully with our understanding of allowing discomfort with equanimity.

Note that patience is different from avoidance. We can be "patient" at the wrong time or in the wrong context. Sometimes we may believe that it is helpful to hold back on taking action, but we are actually avoiding making important decisions. Hence, patience must be weighed against the necessity for immediate action.

## Truthfulness

Truthfulness can be compared to a lantern, always lighting your path even in the darkest nights. When you are truthful with yourself, you dispel confusion, keep a clear mind, and are less likely to worry or catastrophize. If you recall your experiential ownership exercise during interpersonal challenges in week 7, you needed to be honest with yourself about who was responsible for the uncomfortable sensations that co-emerged with your thoughts. In week 8, you equally needed to be truthful during mindful assertiveness in the fourth of the seven statements, stating sincerely "I may be wrong" before asking for what you wanted.

It is equally virtuous to be truthful with others, even though it may sometimes seem that "massaging the truth" will yield a better outcome. You made an effort to be truthful with others during week 9, when you were practicing the use of helpful speech, which includes not misleading others. This involves accepting criticism from others when we recognize it to be true, which helps both parties be more objective about a difficult situation, and allows authenticity to develop in relationships.

## Determination

Determination, or resolve, is the act of committing to what we believe or intend to do. Determination is central to reaching your goals, including resolving family problems, finishing a job or schoolwork on time, staying committed in a relationship, or making the necessary effort to overcome depression and anxiety. However, determination needs to be balanced with wisdom and equanimity, or it can turn into craving, stubbornness, or rigidity. Wisdom and equanimity help prevent going to extremes.

## Kindness

Being kind to yourself and others is an expression of psychological maturity. Kindness is cultivated by the meditation on loving-kindness, which you started practicing in week 9. It is related to compassion, and compassion is related to wisdom—kindness and wisdom are two sides of the same coin. The wiser you become, the kinder you become. This is because remaining kind in the face of someone's challenging expression of their suffering, such as aggressiveness or avoidance, requires a wise understanding of how suffering arises and passes away. Of course, the act of offering kindness is also the act of receiving it. When you are kind toward someone, your kind thoughts co-emerge with pleasant and soothing sensations in the body, and you are the first recipient of your kindness.

## Equanimity

Throughout the book, we have discussed the importance and benefits of cultivating equanimity in your life. Over time, equanimity becomes your best friend. It protects you from agitation and distress as long as you protect it—which you can do by meditating daily. Equanimity is known as one of the four boundless mental states, along with loving-kindness, compassion, and sympathetic joy. Together, these help us cultivate a sense of connection with others and give us a sense of meaning. And a life with meaning is a happier life.

Equanimity is often related to a purity of mind, for good reason (Hart 1987). It is an unconditioned mental state which also has the effect of deconditioning existing mental states—just as a new sponge is free of dirt and has the effect of cleaning the dirt it encounters on its way. When stressful events occur, your ongoing development of equanimity will enable you to see things more objectively.

## Concluding Comments

During the MiCBT program, you used your targeted problems as learning opportunities to develop helpful mental, emotional, and behavioral skills. You then applied and integrated those skills into every aspect of your life. The practice of these skills is a continual process, and you might find it helpful to revisit the concepts in this workbook occasionally. Some people elect to restart the entire program afresh, to benefit from further deepening of the skills.

We hope MiCBT has made a meaningful difference in your life. We equally hope that the benefits you may have gained will also benefit others, especially those you love and care for. We introduced this book with a quote from the poet Ella Wheeler Wilcox, and it seems appropriate to conclude with another (1906):

> *It is easy enough to be pleasant,*
>
> *When life flows by like a song,*
>
> *But the man [sic] worth while is one who will smile,*
>
> *When everything goes dead wrong.*
>
> *For the test of the heart is trouble,*
>
> *And it always comes with the years,*
>
> *And the smile that is worth the praises of earth*
>
> *Is the smile that shines through tears.*
>
> ("Worthwhile," lines 1–8)

---

# Week 10 Checklist

☐  45-minute maintenance practice once daily

☐  Filling in the Equanimity Scale-16 to obtain a post-completion score

# Acknowledgments

We are grateful to Merle Woods, Lorraine Klassen, and Karen Cayoun for their astute feedback on an early draft of this workbook. We are also thankful to Nick Grabovac for his assistance in crafting helpful worksheets, and to the very supportive team at New Harbinger for their guidance. Special appreciation goes to Sally Francis, Alia Offman, and Alice Shires—our shared journeys in teaching and collaborative dialogues have shaped many of the ideas herein.

We are deeply indebted to our principal meditation teachers, S. N. Goenka, Ajahn Jayasaro, and Mahasi Sayadaw, who are part of long lineages of wise teachers who maintained these priceless teachings for nearly twenty-six centuries. Their transformative influence on our own lives is immeasurable. Moreover, we are deeply thankful to our patients and clients over the years. Their trust, insights, and transformative journeys have continually inspired us and reaffirmed the profound impact of these teachings. Our gratitude also flows to our families, who have supported us throughout the writing of this book.

# References

Anālayo. 2018. *Satipatthāna Meditation: A Practice Guide*. Cambridge, UK: Windhorse Publications.

Bauer, C., S. Whitfield-Gabrieli, J. L. Díaz, E. H. Pasaye, and F. A. Barrios. 2019. "From State-to-Trait Meditation: Reconfiguration of Central Executive and Default Mode Networks." *eNeuro* 6(6). https://doi.org/10.1523/ENEURO.0335-18.2019.

Barrett, L. F. 2006. "Valence Is a Basic Building Block of Emotional Life." *Journal of Research in Personality* 40: 35–55. https://doi.org/10.1016/j.jrp.2005.08.006.

Black, D. S., G. A. O'Reilly, R. Olmstead, E. C. Breen, and M. R. Irwin. 2015. "Mindfulness Meditation and Improvement in Sleep Quality and Daytime Impairment Among Older Adults with Sleep Disturbances: A Randomized Clinical Trial." *JAMA Internal Medicine* 175(4): 494–501. https://doi.org/10.1001/jamainternmed.2014.8081.

Bodhi, B. 2005. *In the Buddha's Words: An Anthology of Discourses from the Pali Canon*. Somerville, MA: Wisdom Publications.

Boettcher, H., and D. H. Barlow. 2019. "The Unique and Conditional Effects of Interoceptive Exposure in the Treatment of Anxiety: A functional Analysis." *Behavior Research and Therapy* 117: 65–78. https://doi.org/10.1016/j.brat.2018.12.002.

Cayoun, B., and A. Shires. 2020. "Co-emergence Reinforcement and Its Relevance to Interoceptive Desensitization in Mindfulness and Therapies Aiming at Transdiagnostic Efficacy." *Frontiers in Psychology* 11. https://doi.org/10.3389/fpsyg.2020.545945.

Cayoun, B. A., A. Simmons, and A. Shires. 2020. "Immediate and Lasting Chronic Pain Reduction Following a Brief Self-Implemented Mindfulness-Based Interoceptive Exposure Task: A Pilot Study." *Mindfulness* 11: 112–124. https://doi.org/10.1007/s12671-017-0823-x.

Ecker, B. 2018. "Clinical Translation of Memory Reconsolidation Research: Therapeutic Methodology for Transformational Change by Erasing Implicit Emotional Learnings Driving Symptom Production." *International Journal of Neuropsychotherapy* 6(1): 1–92. https://doi.org/10.12744/ijnpt.2018.0001-0092.

Grabovac, A., M. Lau, and B. Willett. 2011. "Mechanisms of Mindfulness: A Buddhist Psychological Model." *Mindfulness* 2(3): 154–166. https://doi.org/10.1007/s12671-011-0054-5.

Hadash, Y., N. Segev, G. Tanay, P. Goldstein, and A. Bernstein. 2016. "The Decoupling Model of Equanimity: Theory, Measurement, and Test in a Mindfulness Intervention." *Mindfulness* 7(5): 1214–1226. https://psycnet.apa.org/record/2016-35083-001.

Hart, W. 1987. *The Art of Living: Vipassana Meditation as Taught by S. N. Goenka*. New York: Harper & Row.

Holzel, B. K., J. Carmody, K. C. Evans, E. A. Hoge, J. A. Dusek, L. Morgan, R. K. Pitman, and S. W. Lazar. 2010. "Stress Reduction Correlates with Structural Changes in the Amygdala." *Social Cognitive and Affective Neuroscience* 5: 11–17.

Ironside, M., D. C. DeVille, R. T. Kuplicki, K. P. Burrows, R. Smith, A. Teed, M. P. Paulus, and S. S. Khalsa. 2023. "The Unique Face of Comorbid Anxiety and Depression: Increased Interoceptive Fearfulness and Reactivity." *Frontiers in Behavioural Neuroscience* 16. https://doi.org/10.3389/fnbeh.2022.1083357.

Jacobson, E. 1942. *You Must Relax*. New York: McGraw-Hill.

Jayasaro, A. 2010. "The Paramis as Practices of Liberation." Amaravati Buddhist Monastery, May 22. Accessed August 28, 2023. https://amaravati.org/audio/the-paramis-as-practices-of-liberation-ajahn-jayasaro-22052010.

Joyce, J. 1914. *Dubliners*. London: Grant Richards.

Juneau, C., N. Pellerin, T. Elliott, M. Ricard, R. Shankland, and M. Dambrun. 2020. "Reliability and Validity of an Equanimity Questionnaire: The Two-Factor Equanimity Scale (EQUA-S)." *PeerJ* 8(e9405): 1–19. https://doi.org/10.7717/peerj.9405.

Khalsa, S. S., R. Adolphs, O. G. Cameron, H. D. Critchley, P. W. Davenport, J. S. Feinstein, et al. 2018. "Interoception and Mental Health: A Roadmap." *Biological Psychiatry Cognitive Neuroscience and Neuroimaging* 3: 501–513. https://doi: 10.1016/j.bpsc.2017.12.004.

Möller, H., B. Bandelow, H-P. Volz, U. Barnikol, E. Seifritz, and S. Kasper. 2016. "The Relevance of 'Mixed Anxiety and Depression' as a Diagnostic Category in Clinical Practice." *European Archives of Psychiatry and Clinical Neuroscience* 266(8): 725–736.

Nummenmaa, L., E. Glerean, R. Hari, and J. K. Hietanen. 2013. "Bodily Maps of Emotions." *Proceedings of the National Academy of Sciences of the USA* 111(2): 646–651. https://doi.org/10.1073/pnas.1321664111.

Rogers, H., A. Shires, B. Cayoun. 2021. "Development and Validation of the Equanimity Scale-16." *Mindfulness* 12(2): 1–14. https://doi.org/10.1007/s12671-020-01503-6.

Shires, A., S. Osborne, B. A. Cayoun, E. Williams, and K. Rogers. 2023. "Predictive Validity and Response Shift in the Equanimity Scale-16." *Mindfulness* 14: 2880–2893. https://doi.org/10.1007/s12671-023-02257-7.

ter Avest, M. J., R. Schuling, C. U. Greven, M. J. Huijbers, T. F. Wilderjans, P. Spinhoven, and A. E. M. Speckens. 2021. "Interplay Between Self-Compassion and Affect During Mindfulness-Based Compassionate Living for Recurrent Depression: An Autoregressive Latent Trajectory Analysis." *Behaviour Research and Therapy* 146: 103946. https://doi.org/10.1016/j.brat.2021.103946.

Varela, F. J., E. Thompson, and E. Rosch. 1991. *The Embodied Mind: Cognitive Science and Human Experience*. Cambridge, MA: MIT Press.

Wilcox, E. W. 1883. *Poems of Passion*. Chicago: W. B. Conkey Co.

———. 1906. *Poems of Sentiment*. Chicago: W. B. Conkey Co.

Wu, Q., X. Mao, W. Luo, J. Fan, X. Liu, and Y. Wu. 2022. "Enhanced Interoceptive Attention Mediates the Relationship Between Mindfulness Training and the Reduction of Negative Mood." *Psychophysiology* 59: e13991. https://doi.org/10.1111/psyp.13991.

**Andrea D. Grabovac, MD,** is a clinical psychiatrist practicing in Vancouver, Canada. She is codirector of the North American chapter of the MiCBT Institute, and is clinical professor of psychiatry at the University of British Columbia. With over twenty-five years of clinical experience, she trains mental health clinicians locally and internationally in the delivery of MiCBT and mindfulness-based cognitive therapy (MBCT). Grabovac is continually involved in mindfulness research, developing competency-based mindfulness training approaches, and regularly publishes in scientific journals. She practices mindfulness meditation in the Burmese Theravada tradition, and is a certified yoga teacher. She is coauthor of the *Mindfulness for Men* course, available on the HeadsUpGuys website.

**Bruno A. Cayoun, DPsych, MACPA,** is a clinical and research psychologist, and principal developer of mindfulness-integrated cognitive behavior therapy (MiCBT). He is director of the MiCBT Institute, the leading provider of MiCBT training and professional development to mental health services and professional associations internationally since 2003. Cayoun has practiced mindfulness meditation in the Burmese Vipassana tradition of S. N. Goenka since 1989. He has kept a private psychology practice in Hobart, Australia, implementing MiCBT with groups and individuals with a wide range of mental health difficulties for the past twenty years. He is author of several book chapters and books, including *Mindfulness-integrated CBT, Mindfulness-integrated CBT for Well-Being and Personal Growth,* and is coauthor of *The Clinical Handbook of Mindfulness-integrated Cognitive Behavior Therapy.*

# MORE BOOKS from
# NEW HARBINGER PUBLICATIONS

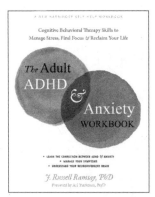
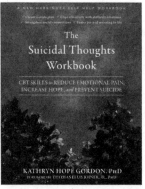
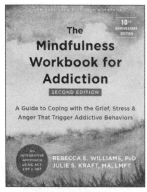
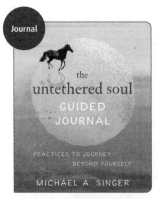
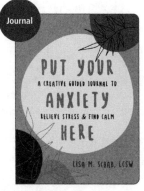
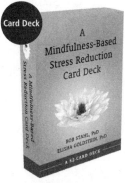

# Did you know there are **free tools** you can download for this book?

Free tools are things like **worksheets**, **guided meditation exercises**, and **more** that will help you get the most out of your book.

You can download free tools for this book—whether you bought or borrowed it, in any format, from any source—from the New Harbinger website. All you need is a NewHarbinger.com account. Just use the URL provided in this book to view the free tools that are available for it. Then, click on the "download" button for the free tool you want, and follow the prompts that appear to log in to your NewHarbinger.com account and download the material.

You can also save the free tools for this book to your **Free Tools Library** so you can access them again anytime, just by logging in to your account! Just look for this button on the book's free tools page.

**+ Save this to my free tools library**